From Menarche to Menopause:
The Female Body
in Feminist Therapy

From Menarche to Menopause: The Female Body in Feminist Therapy has been co-published simultaneously as *Women & Therapy*, Volume 27, Numbers 3/4 2004.

The *Women & Therapy* Monographic "Separates"

Below is a list of "separates," which in serials librarianship means a special issue simultaneously published as a special journal issue or double-issue *and* as a "separate" hardbound monograph. (This is a format which we also call a "DocuSerial.")

"Separates" are published because specialized libraries or professionals may wish to purchase a specific thematic issue by itself in a format which can be separately cataloged and shelved, as opposed to purchasing the journal on an on-going basis. Faculty members may also more easily consider a "separate" for classroom adoption.

"Separates" are carefully classified separately with the major book jobbers so that the journal tie-in can be noted on new book order slips to avoid duplicate purchasing.

You may wish to visit Haworth's website at . . .

http://www.HaworthPress.com

. . . to search our online catalog for complete tables of contents of these separates and related publications.

You may also call 1-800-HAWORTH (outside US/Canada: 607-722-5857), or Fax 1-800-895-0582 (outside US/Canada: 607-771-0012), or e-mail at:

docdelivery@haworthpress.com

From Menarche to Menopause: The Female Body in Feminist Therapy, edited by Joan C. Chrisler, PhD (Vol. 27, No. 3/4, 2004). *"A definitive resource on women's reproductive health. . . . Brings this topic out of the closet. . . . The coverage is excellent, spanning the adolescent experience of menarche and moving from pregnancy issues to menopause and beyond. The chapter authors are clearly experts on their topics, and this edited book is admirable in its philosophical coherence. Feminist therapists working with young girls, women in their reproductive years, and older women will find clear information about how to understand and affirm their clients' experiences." (Maryka Biaggio, PhD, Professor and Director of Research on Feminist Issues, Department of Professional Psychiatry, Pacific University)*

Biracial Women in Therapy: Between the Rock of Gender and the Hard Place of Race, edited by Angela R. Gillem, PhD, and Cathy A. Thompson, PhD (Vol. 27, No. 1/2, 2004). *"A must-read. . . . Compelling and poignant. . . . Enhances our understanding of what it means to be biracial and female in society dominated by monoracial notions of identity and sexualized notions of biracial women. . . . Delves insightfully into a variety of biracial women's experiences." (Lisa Bowleg, PhD, Assistant Professor, Department of Psychology, University of Rhode Island)*

Women with Visible and Invisible Disabilities: Multiple Intersections, Multiple Issues, Multiple Therapies, edited by Martha E. Banks, PhD, and Ellyn Kaschak, PhD (Vol. 26, No. 1/2/3/4, 2003). *"Bravo . . . provides powerful and direct answers to the questions, concerns, and challenges all women with disability experience. The voices in this book are speaking loud and clear to a wide range of readers and audiences. . . . Centered on the core principle that quality of life revolves around one's mental health, a sense of strength, and resiliency." (Theresa M. Rankin, BA, NCE, National Community Educator, Brain Injury Services, Inc.; MidAtlantic Traumatic Brain Injury Consortium; Fairhaven Institute for Brain Injury/University of Wisconsin-Scott)*

Violence in the Lives of Black Women: Battered, Black, and Blue, edited by Carolyn M. West, PhD (Vol. 25, No. 3/4, 2002). *Helps break the silence surrounding Black women's experiences of violence.*

Exercise and Sport in Feminist Therapy: Constructing Modalities and Assessing Outcomes, edited by Ruth L. Hall, PhD, and Carole A. Oglesby, PhD (Vol. 25, No. 2, 2002). *Explores the healing use of exercise and sport as a helpful adjunct to feminist therapy.*

The Invisible Alliance: Psyche and Spirit in Feminist Therapy, edited by Ellyn Kaschak, PhD (Vol. 24, No. 3/4, 2001). *"The richness of this volume is reflected in the diversity of the collected viewpoints, perspectives, and practices. Each chapter challenges us to move out of the confines of our traditional training and reflect on the importance of spirituality. This book also brings us back to the original meaning of psychology–the study and knowledge of the soul." (Stephanie S. Covington, PhD, LCSW, Co-Director, Institute for Relational Development, La Jolla, California; Author, A Woman's Way Through the Twelve Steps)*

A New View of Women's Sexual Problems, edited by Ellyn Kaschak, PhD, and Leonore Tiefer, PhD (Vol. 24, No. 1/2, 2001). *"This useful, complex, and valid critique of simplistic notions of women's sexuality will be especially valuable for women's studies and public health courses. An important compilation representing many diverse individuals and groups of women." (Judy Norsigian and Jane Pincus, Co-Founders, Boston Women's Health Collective; Co-Authors,* Our Bodies, Ourselves for the New Century)

Intimate Betrayal: Domestic Violence in Lesbian Relationships, edited by Ellyn Kaschak, PhD (Vol. 23, No. 3, 2001). *"A groundbreaking examination of a taboo and complex subject. Both scholarly and down to earth, this superbly edited volume is an indispensable resource for clinicians, researchers, and lesbians caught up in the cycle of domestic violence." (Dr. Marny Hall, Psychotherapist; Author of* The Lesbian Love Companion, *Co-Author of* Queer Blues)

The Next Generation: Third Wave Feminist Psychotherapy, edited by Ellyn Kaschak, PhD (Vol. 23, No. 2, 2001). *Discusses the issues young feminists face, focusing on the implications for psychotherapists of the false sense that feminism is no longer necessary.*

Minding the Body: Psychotherapy in Cases of Chronic and Life-Threatening Illness, edited by Ellyn Kaschak, PhD (Vol. 23, No. 1, 2001). *Being diagnosed with cancer, lupus, or fibromyalgia is a traumatic event. All too often, women are told their disease is "all in their heads" and, therefore, both "unreal and insignificant" by a medical profession that dismisses emotions and scorns mental illness. Combining personal narratives and theoretical views of illness,* Minding the Body *offers an alternative approach to the mind-body connection. This book shows the reader how to deal with the painful and difficult emotions that exacerbate illness, while learning the emotional and spiritual lessons illness can teach.*

For Love or Money: The Fee in Feminist Therapy, edited by Marcia Hill, EdD, and Ellyn Kaschak, PhD (Vol. 22, No. 3, 1999). *"Recommended reading for both new and seasoned professionals. . . . An exciting and timely book about 'the last taboo.' . . ." (Carolyn C. Larsen, PhD, Senior Counsellor Emeritus, University of Calgary; Partner, Alberta Psychological Resources Ltd., Calgary, and Co-Editor,* Ethical Decision Making in Therapy: Feminist Perspectives)

Beyond the Rule Book: Moral Issues and Dilemmas in the Practice of Psychotherapy, edited by Ellyn Kaschak, PhD, and Marcia Hill, EdD (Vol. 22, No. 2, 1999). *"The authors in this important and timely book tackle the difficult task of working through . . . conflicts, sharing their moral struggles and real life solutions in working with diverse populations and in a variety of clinical settings. . . . Will provide psychotherapists with a thought-provoking source for the stimulating and essential discussion of our own and our profession's moral bases." (Carolyn C. Larsen, PhD, Senior Counsellor Emeritus, University of Calgary, Partner in private practice, Alberta Psychological Resources Ltd., Calgary, and Co-Editor,* Ethical Decision Making in Therapy: Feminist Perspectives)

Assault on the Soul: Women in the Former Yugoslavia, edited by Sara Sharratt, PhD, and Ellyn Kaschak, PhD (Vol. 22, No. 1, 1999). *Explores the applications and intersections of feminist therapy, activism and jurisprudence with women and children in the former Yugoslavia.*

Learning from Our Mistakes: Difficulties and Failures in Feminist Therapy, edited by Marcia Hill, EdD, and Esther D. Rothblum, PhD (Vol. 21, No. 3, 1998). *"A courageous and fundamental step in evolving a well-grounded body of theory and of investigating the assumptions that, unexamined, lead us to error." (Teresa Bernardez, MD, Training and Supervising Analyst, The Michigan Psychoanalytic Council)*

Feminist Therapy as a Political Act, edited by Marcia Hill, EdD (Vol. 21, No. 2, 1998). *"A real contribution to the field. . . . A valuable tool for feminist therapists and those who want to learn about feminist therapy." (Florence L. Denmark, PhD, Robert S. Pace, Distinguished Professor of Psychology and Chair, Psychology Department, Pace University, New York, New York)*

Breaking the Rules: Women in Prison and Feminist Therapy, edited by Judy Harden, PhD, and Marcia Hill, EdD (Vol. 20, No. 4 & Vol. 21, No. 1, 1998). *"Fills a long-recognized gap in the psychology of women curricula, demonstrating that feminist theory can be made relevant to the practice of feminism, even in prison." (Suzanne J. Kessler, PhD, Professor of Psychology and Women's Studies, State University of New York at Purchase)*

Children's Rights, Therapists' Responsibilities: Feminist Commentaries, edited by Gail Anderson, MA, and Marcia Hill, EdD (Vol. 20, No. 2, 1997). *"Addresses specific practice dimensions that will help therapists organize and resolve conflicts about working with children, adolescents, and their families in therapy." (Feminist Bookstore News)*

More than a Mirror: How Clients Influence Therapists' Lives, edited by Marcia Hill, EdD (Vol. 20, No. 1, 1997). *"Courageous, insightful, and deeply moving. These pages reveal the scrupulous self-examination and self-reflection of conscientious therapists at their best. An important contribution to feminist therapy literature and a book worth reading by therapists and clients alike." (Rachel Josefowitz Siegal, MSW, retired feminist therapy practitioner; Co-Editor,* Women Changing Therapy; Jewish Women in Therapy; *and* Celebrating the Lives of Jewish Women: Patterns in a Feminist Sampler)

Sexualities, edited by Marny Hall, PhD, LCSW (Vol. 19, No. 4, 1997). *"Explores the diverse and multifaceted nature of female sexuality, covering topics including sadomasochism in the therapy room, sexual exploitation in cults, and genderbending in cyberspace." (Feminist Bookstore News)*

Couples Therapy: Feminist Perspectives, edited by Marcia Hill, EdD, and Esther D. Rothblum, PhD (Vol. 19, No. 3, 1996). *Addresses some of the inadequacies, omissions, and assumptions in traditional couples' therapy to help you face the issues of race, ethnicity, and sexual orientation in helping couples today.*

A Feminist Clinician's Guide to the Memory Debate, edited by Susan Contratto, PhD, and M. Janice Gutfreund, PhD (Vol. 19, No. 1, 1996). *"Unites diverse scholars, clinicians, and activists in an insightful and useful examination of the issues related to recovered memories." (Feminist Bookstore News)*

Classism and Feminist Therapy: Counting Costs, edited by Marcia Hill, EdD, and Esther D. Rothblum, PhD (Vol. 18, No. 3/4, 1996). *"Educates, challenges, and questions the influence of classism on the clinical practice of psychotherapy with women." (Kathleen P. Gates, MA, Certified Professional Counselor, Center for Psychological Health, Superior, Wisconsin)*

Lesbian Therapists and Their Therapy: From Both Sides of the Couch, edited by Nancy D. Davis, MD, Ellen Cole, PhD, and Esther D. Rothblum, PhD (Vol. 18, No. 2, 1996). *"Highlights the power and boundary issues of psychotherapy from perspectives that many readers may have neither considered nor experienced in their own professional lives." (Psychiatric Services)*

Feminist Foremothers in Women's Studies, Psychology, and Mental Health, edited by Phyllis Chesler, PhD, Esther D. Rothblum, PhD, and Ellen Cole, PhD (Vol. 17, No. 1/2/3/4, 1995). *"A must for feminist scholars and teachers . . . These women's personal experiences are poignant and powerful." (Women's Studies International Forum)*

Women's Spirituality, Women's Lives, edited by Judith Ochshorn, PhD, and Ellen Cole, PhD (Vol. 16, No. 2/3, 1995). *"A delightful and complex book on spirituality and sacredness in women's lives." (Joan Clingan, MA, Spiritual Psychology, Graduate Advisor, Prescott College Master of Arts Program)*

Psychopharmacology from a Feminist Perspective, edited by Jean A. Hamilton, MD, Margaret Jensvold, MD, Esther D. Rothblum, PhD, and Ellen Cole, PhD (Vol. 16, No. 1, 1995). *"Challenges readers to increase their sensitivity and awareness of the role of sex and gender in response to and acceptance of pharmacologic therapy." (American Journal of Pharmaceutical Education)*

Wilderness Therapy for Women: The Power of Adventure, edited by Ellen Cole, PhD, Esther D. Rothblum, PhD, and Eve Erdman, MEd, MLS (Vol. 15, No. 3/4, 1994). *"There's an undeniable excitement in these pages about the thrilling satisfaction of meeting challenges in the physical world, the world outside our cities that is unfamiliar, uneasy territory for many women. If you're interested at all in the subject, this book is well worth your time." (Psychology of Women Quarterly)*

Bringing Ethics Alive: Feminist Ethics in Psychotherapy Practice, edited by Nanette K. Gartrell, MD (Vol. 15, No. 1, 1994). *"Examines the theoretical and practical issues of ethics in feminist therapies. From the responsibilities of training programs to include social issues ranging from racism to sexism to practice ethics, this outlines real questions and concerns." (Midwest Book Review)*

Women with Disabilities: Found Voices, edited by Mary Willmuth, PhD, and Lillian Holcomb, PhD (Vol. 14, No. 3/4, 1994). *"These powerful chapters often jolt the anti-disability consciousness and force readers to contend with the ways in which disability has been constructed, disguised, and rendered disgusting by much of society." (Academic Library Book Review)*

Faces of Women and Aging, edited by Nancy D. Davis, MD, Ellen Cole, PhD, and Esther D. Rothblum, PhD (Vol. 14, No. 1/2, 1993). *"This uplifting, helpful book is of great value not only for aging women, but also for women of all ages who are interested in taking active control of their own lives." (New Mature Woman)*

Monographs "Separates" list continued at the back

From Menarche to Menopause: The Female Body in Feminist Therapy

Joan C. Chrisler, PhD
Editor

From Menarche to Menopause: The Female Body in Feminist Therapy has been co-published simultaneously as *Women & Therapy*, Volume 27, Numbers 3/4 2004.

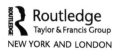

Routledge
Taylor & Francis Group
NEW YORK AND LONDON

First published by
The Haworth Press, Inc.
10 Alice Street
Binghamton, N Y 13904-1580

This edition published 2011 by Routledge

Routledge
Taylor & Francis Group
711 Third Avenue
New York, NY 10017

Routledge
Taylor & Francis Group
2 Park Square, Milton Park
Abingdon, Oxon OX14 4RN

From Menarche to Menopause: The Female Body in Feminist Therapy has been co-published simultaneously as *Women & Therapy*, Volume 27, Numbers 3/4 2004.

Cover design by Jennifer M. Gaska

Library of Congress Cataloging-in-Publication Data

From menarche to menopause : the female body in feminist therapy / Joan C. Chrisler, editor.
    p. cm.
    "Co-published simultaneously as Women & Therapy, vol. 27, no. 3/4 2004."
    Includes bibliographical references and index.
    ISBN 0-7890-2349-0 (hbk. : alk. paper) – ISBN 0-7890-2350-4 (pbk. : alk. paper)
    1. Feminist therapy. 2. Menarche. 3. Menopause. 4. Body image. I. Chrisler, Joan C.
II. Women & therapy.
RC489.F45F76 2003
616.89′14–dc22   2003018226

From Menarche to Menopause: The Female Body in Feminist Therapy

CONTENTS

ABOUT THE EDITOR

Joan C. Chrisler, PhD, is Professor of Psychology at Connecticut College in New London, Connecticut, where she teaches courses on the psychology of women and health psychology. She has published dozens of journal articles and book chapters on women's health, and she is particularly known for her work on menstruation and menopause, autoimmune disorders, body image, weight, and eating disorders. She has edited special issues of *Women's Studies Quarterly, Sex Roles,* and *Women & Health,* and has edited several books, including *New Directions in Feminist Psychology, Charting a New Course for Feminist Psychology, Variations on a Theme: Diversity and the Psychology of Women, Lectures on the Psychology of Women,* and *Arming Athena: Career Strategies for Women in Academe.*

Introduction

Joan C. Chrisler

Are you surprised to see a volume of *Women & Therapy* about *including* women's bodies in the therapy context? Thirty years ago the focus of a collection such as this would have been on the necessity of *excluding* topics such as menstruation, pregnancy, and menopause from diagnosis and deliberation. Early feminist therapists, researchers, and theorists were actively engaged in gathering data and constructing arguments against sexist notions that women's bodies were essentially defective and the cause of women's mental, as well as physical, suffering.

As a psychology student I was taught that menstruation caused all manner of physical ailments and mental anguish, that women often "went crazy" after giving birth or during the menopausal transition, that rejection of femininity led to dysmenorrhea and infertility, and that many issues connected to women's reproductive systems (perhaps especially menarche and miscarriage) were best left unmentioned in both personal and professional conversations. I was also taught that pregnancy would cure many of women's problems, including dysmenorrhea and depression. (Oddly, the fact that pregnancy leads to birth, which we were told leads to depression, was never mentioned. Were women expected to stay pregnant all the time in order to preserve their mental health?) Second wave feminists were kept busy with the task of normalizing and de-stigmatizing women's bodily functions and pointing out that cultural pressures, social constructions, and neurochemical processes had as much or more to do with women's mental health than did reproductive status. Although it is not impossible to find people who still believe the statements above, it is safe to say that progress has been made. The average psychotherapist no longer immediately assumes that a woman is angry because she is premenstrual or that a woman is infertile because she hates her female body.

[Haworth co-indexing entry note]: "Introduction." Chrisler, Joan C. Co-published simultaneously in *Women & Therapy* (The Haworth Press, Inc.) Vol. 27, No. 3/4, 2004, pp. 1-3; and: *From Menarche to Menopause: The Female Body in Feminist Therapy* (ed: Joan C. Chrisler) The Haworth Press, Inc., 2004, pp. 1-3. Single or multiple copies of this article are available for a fee from The Haworth Document Delivery Service [1-800-HAWORTH, 9:00 a.m. - 5:00 p.m. (EST). E-mail address: docdelivery@haworthpress.com].

http://www.haworthpress.com/store/product.asp?sku=J015
10.1300/J015v27n03_01

This is not to suggest that women's bodies have been ignored by feminist therapists and theorists. Many conversations about bodies take place in the therapeutic context. However, the focus of therapists, researchers, and theorists has been on the outside of the body rather than the inside, physique rather than physiology. Frequent topics in feminist discourse are body weight, body dissatisfaction, and body dysphoria. Many women enter therapy to talk about eating disorders, body image, and appearance anxiety. In recent years attempts have been made to broaden the range of body topics that can be dealt with in feminist therapy. *Women & Therapy* has been a leader in this effort by publishing special issues on such body-related topics as aging, chronic illness, and physical activity.

It is time for a more sophisticated perspective on the female body and the ways that living in one affects women's experiences. Women do bleed, birth, and flash. Some get pregnant when they don't want to, and others don't get pregnant when they do want to. Some pregnancies result in joy; others result in sorrow. Some births are exciting and empowering; others are disappointing and disempowering. Some women have mild menstrual and menopausal symptoms; others have moderate or severe symptoms that interfere with their social and professional lives. Many women have been harmed by the silence and stigma that surrounds infertility, menarche, miscarriage, and menopause. Body image, gender identity, and self-acceptance are a few of the many factors that can be affected by the reproductive processes of the female body. If these factors can be discussed in feminist therapy, why not also discuss the physiological processes that provide part of the context of the experience?

There is a large literature on each of the topics discussed in this collection, and a busy psychotherapist cannot possibly read, much less master, them all. Thus, each author in this volume was given the task of reviewing the most important empirical, theoretical, and political work on her topic so that a reader can quickly grasp the main issues. In addition, each author suggests ways that therapists can approach the topic in treatment, and many offer bibliotherapy and Internet resources that can be suggested to clients who want to learn more about the topics. Clients may often come to therapy with established beliefs based on myths (such as those I was taught in college) that were passed on to them by family, friends, professors, or physicians or that are based on inaccurate information they've picked up from the media. A recent "hot topic" in the media is the notion that menstruating is bad for women's health and should be suppressed except when a woman wants to become pregnant. Those media stories were drawn from publicity for a book titled *Is Menstruation Obsolete?* (Coutinho & Segal, 1999), which is reviewed in this volume. The authors of the papers included herein provide assistance in counteracting much of the myth and misinformation that clients (and therapists themselves) may have heard.

We see our work on this volume as a service to feminist therapists and, frankly, as a labor of love–because most of us have committed the bulk of our scholarship to work on women's reproductive health. Who are we? Most of the authors are members of the Society for Menstrual Cycle Research, which was incorporated in 1979, and was the first multidisciplinary group that actively promoted research on women's health. The founding members realized that menstruation is a gender-specific process that had rarely been studied outside of its reproductive potential and usually only in a negative light. Since 1977 the Society has sponsored biennial conferences, which have resulted in more than a dozen published volumes of research on menstruation, menopause, and related aspects of women's health. The Society publishes a quarterly newsletter as well as books, conference proceedings, and special issues of journals. We also serve as an important forum for collaboration among biomedical, behavioral, and social scientists; humanists; public policy advocates; and health care providers. Although other women's health organizations have emerged in recent years, the Society remains committed to providing an interdisciplinary focus that is rare elsewhere. Our international membership includes leaders in women's health research, education, practice, policy, and advocacy. Most presentations at our conferences are explicitly feminist in their approach, and we have often joined activist coalitions to promote public policy or awareness of women's health issues. To learn more about the Society, please visit our Web site at <www.pop.psu.edu/smcr>.

Menarche and menopause are perhaps the only topics in this volume that *all* women experience; however, the fact that we *could* experience all of the topics is a major contributor to our identity as women. Although only a few of the topics (e.g., premenstrual or childbearing depression; grief due to miscarriage, stillbirth, or infertility) are likely to, of themselves, cause women to seek psychotherapy, any of the topics may be raised in therapy by women who have sought treatment for other reasons. Thus it is useful for therapists who work with women to have some knowledge of the topics and easy access to lists of references and resources should further knowledge be needed. We sincerely hope that our work will aid our readers in their work.

Self-Objectification
and That "Not So Fresh Feeling":
Feminist Therapeutic Interventions
for Healthy Female Embodiment

Tomi-Ann Roberts
Patricia L. Waters

SUMMARY. In a culture obsessed with women's attractiveness and beauty, media messages abound telling us our corporeal bodies are unacceptable as they are. Women's bodies need sanitizing, deodorizing, exfoliating, and denuding. Perhaps more than any other bodily function, menstruation must be kept "under wraps" in a sexually objectifying culture. In this article, we argue that girls' and women's feelings of accep-

Tomi-Ann Roberts is Associate Professor of Psychology at Colorado College. She received her PhD in social and personality psychology from Stanford University in 1990. Her research focuses on the social construction of the body and objectification theory. Patricia L. Waters is Assistant Professor of Psychology at Colorado College. She received her PhD in developmental psychology from Boston University in 1991, and completed postdoc and clinical training at the University of Denver. Her research interests lie in adolescence, depression, and voice. Both Roberts and Waters are active teachers, scholars, and mentors in Colorado College's interdisciplinary Women's Studies program.

Address correspondence to: Tomi-Ann Roberts and Patricia L. Waters, Department of Psychology, Colorado College, Colorado Springs, CO 80903 (E-mail: troberts@coloradocollege.edu).

[Haworth co-indexing entry note]: "Self-Objectification and That 'Not So Fresh Feeling': Feminist Therapeutic Interventions for Healthy Female Embodiment." Roberts, Tomi-Ann, and Patricia L. Waters. Co-published simultaneously in *Women & Therapy* (The Haworth Press, Inc.) Vol. 27, No. 3/4, 2004, pp. 5-21; and: *From Menarche to Menopause: The Female Body in Feminist Therapy* (ed: Joan C. Chrisler) The Haworth Press, Inc., 2004, pp. 5-21. Single or multiple copies of this article are available for a fee from The Haworth Document Delivery Service [1-800-HAWORTH, 9:00 a.m. - 5:00 p.m. (EST). E-mail address: docdelivery@haworthpress.com].

10.1300/J015v27n03_02

tance for their bodily functions and physical embodiment are antithetical to "self-objectification," wherein individuals internalize an outsider's standard of physical appearance. We further argue that objectification theory can inform a feminist framework for therapists to use to help clients cope with a particular kind of self-loathing–disgust and shame about their physical selves, including their menstrual periods, in a culture that values impossibly idealized feminine embodiment. *[Article copies available for a fee from The Haworth Document Delivery Service: 1-800-HAWORTH. E-mail address: <docdelivery@haworthpress.com> Website: <http://www.HaworthPress.com> © 2004 by The Haworth Press, Inc. All rights reserved.]*

KEYWORDS. Objectification, menstruation, shame, disgust, embodiment

A frantic mother of a 18-year-old daughter posted a disconcerting letter to an Internet listserv. In it she sought advice as to whether she should agree to allow her daughter to undergo a voluntary hysterectomy. Apparently her child was so ashamed and disgusted by her menstrual periods that during them she confined herself to the home. Her feelings of self-disgust were so overwhelming that she felt she could not face others. Her periods made her feel like an "untouchable"–ugly and repulsive at a time in life when her attractiveness to others, and especially to men, was of utmost importance to her self-esteem. What she wanted, more than anything, was to be rid of her monthly befouling menstrual ordeal entirely so that she could feel attractive and socially desirable. A hysterectomy appeared to her to be the best solution. Was it ethical, the mother asked the listserv members, to agree to allow a doctor to remove the reproductive organs of her perfectly healthy daughter? If it would truly provide a solution to her depression and monthly self-imposed quarantine, would it in fact be *the* ethical thing to do?

In a culture obsessed with women's attractiveness and beauty, media messages abound telling us our corporeal bodies are unacceptable as they are. Women's bodies need sanitizing, deodorizing, exfoliating, and denuding. Perhaps more than any other bodily function, menstruation must be kept "under wraps" in a sexually objectifying culture. Although no longer confined to menstrual huts, Western women must nevertheless conceal menstruation. The marketing of menstrual hygiene or management products emphasizes an ideal of super-femininity, modesty, and decorum (Coutts & Berg, 1993) and promises young women a sanitized, deodorized, and "fresh" bodily presentation. Of course men are the most important people from whom to conceal evidence of menstruation. Countless advertisements are designed to induce anxiety that men might *find out*; these ads imply that such revelation would mean a devastating decrease of a woman's attractiveness and popularity. For example, in a *Pursettes* advertisement from the 1970s in which a teenaged girl drops a tampon out of her bag, the copy reads: "I spilled my secret and he almost found out!" (courtesy of the Museum of Menstruation, www.mum.org). Fortunately, *Pursettes* are specifically designed to be small enough generally to go unnoticed, even if dropped!

In this article, we argue that an 18-year-old's desire for a hysterectomy, although disturbing, is perhaps not mystifying. From the perspective of objectification theory (Fredrickson & Roberts, 1997), feelings of acceptance for one's bodily functions and physical embodiment are antithetical to "self-objectification," wherein individuals internalize an outsider's standard of physical appearance. We further argue that objectification theory can inform a feminist framework for therapists to use to help clients cope with a particular kind of self-loathing–disgust and shame about their physical selves, including their menstrual periods, in a culture that values impossibly idealized feminine embodiment.

OBJECTIFICATION THEORY

A number of feminist theorists (e.g., Kaschak, 1992; Ussher, 1989) have argued that, in a culture in which the sexualized evaluation of girls' and women's bodies is normative, girls and women can come to treat themselves on some level as objects to be looked at and evaluated. That is, women learn, both directly and vicariously, that their "looks" matter, that other people's evaluations of their physical appearance can determine how they are treated, and, ultimately, these evaluations affect their social and economic life outcomes. Objectification theory (Fredrickson & Roberts, 1997), which owes its roots to feminist thinkers such as de Beauvoir (1952), Young (1990), and Kaschak (1992), articulates a host of psychological consequences of the sexual objectification of women and argues that women can adopt a "third-person" or "looking-glass" perspective on their physical selves as a way of anticipating and controlling their treatment–an effect termed "self-objectification"–which may in part supplant a more "first-person" point-of-view. Thus an "outside-in" perspective dominates over an "inside-out" one.

Self-objectification is theorized to lead to a variety of emotional and behavioral costs, which researchers have begun to demonstrate (e.g., Fredrickson, Roberts, Noll, Quinn, & Twenge, 1998; McKinley & Hyde, 1996; Noll & Fredrickson, 1998). First and foremost, it leads to a form of self-consciousness that is characterized by a preoccupation with the body's outward appearance as opposed to its health or functioning. This preoccupation is theorized to demand cognitive resources, and indeed has been shown to disrupt women's, but not men's, cognitive performance on demanding concurrent activities (Fredrickson et al., 1998). Self-objectification has also been shown to lead to negative emotions such as shame, disgust, and anxiety for women but not men (e.g., Fredrickson et al., 1998; Roberts, Gettman, Konik, & Fredrickson, 2000). Finally, accumulations of negative emotions that stem from self-objectification are theorized to contribute to a variety of mental and physical problems experienced predominantly by women, such as eating disorders and depression (Fredrickson & Roberts, 1997).

Research shows that individuals differ in the extent to which they self-objectify; women overall do so more than men, but there is considerable variation among women themselves (e.g., Fredrickson et al., 1998; McKinley & Hyde, 1996). Furthermore, objectification theory predicts a developmental course for self-objectification and its attendant psychological consequences. This perspective on bodily self is hypothesized to begin at puberty, when maturational changes in the body are experienced within the context of increasing sexualized attention and evaluative commentary (e.g., Martin, 1996), and may end at midlife to the extent that women, within a culture that equates aging with decreased sexual desirability, are more willing and able to step out of the objectification limelight. Indeed cross-sectional research has shown that younger women, regardless of ethnicity, show higher levels of self-objectification than do older women (e.g., Roberts, 2000).

HISTORICAL CONCEPTIONS
OF WOMEN'S BODILY INFERIORITY

Historically, and across a wide array of cultures, attitudes toward women have emphasized their bodily connection to nature (see Tauna, 1993). Philosophical and religious perspectives in patriarchal societies have long stressed the "mind" and "soul" as the defining characteristics that elevate human beings above the status of animals. Within these frameworks women have been viewed, in contrast to men, as being ruled by their physical bodies and bodily functions (e.g., de Beauvoir, 1952). For example, Aristotle (1984) argued that women's inferiority to men was tied specifically to menstrual blood, which he viewed as less pure than the semen of men. Freud (1918/1964) wrote that women's inherent inferiority to men is rooted in their reproductive biology, which they cannot sublimate or "civilize" as fully as men can.

There is much anthropological evidence that women's menstruation especially has been feared, denigrated, and subjected to cultural taboos (see Delaney, Lupton, & Toth, 1988). From the Bible to the Koran, injunctions against contact with women during menstruation illustrate the cultural belief that women are polluting and that menstrual blood can have a contaminating effect. Many cultures confined women to menstrual huts, or required ritual baths following menstruation, in order to ensure men's safety from contact. Taboos restricting contact by menstruating women with food and with men remained in many cultures well into the 19th century, and have continued in some cultures into the 21st century (Delaney et al., 1988; Slonim, 1996; Whelan, 1975). There continues to be evidence that menstruating women are perceived as polluting, through for example, the wide endorsement of myths such as those dictating that women should not have intercourse during menstruation (*The Tampax Report*, 1981). Although

Western women do not confine themselves to menstrual huts, advertisers certainly market menstruation as a "hygiene crisis" that must be concealed and managed with products that enable women to avoid staining, soiling, odor, and humiliation (Havens & Swenson, 1988). Indeed research shows that many contemporary women are anxious about being "discovered," and thus humiliated, through odor or staining their clothes (Kissling, 1996; Lee, 1994; Ussher, 1989). Lee (1994) has argued that staining is a visible emblem of women's contamination and supposed bodily inferiority, and it symbolizes a lapse in the culturally mandated responsibility of all women to conceal evidence of menstruation.

OBJECTIFICATION OF WOMEN AS CULTURAL DEFENSE AGAINST WOMEN'S CORPOREAL BODIES

The findings from recent research (Roberts, Goldenberg, Power, & Pyszczynski, 2002) illustrate the great lengths to which many women go to avoid revelation of menstrual status and discussion of related issues. In this study, both men and women exhibited negative reactions to a woman who inadvertently dropped a wrapped tampon out of her bag. She was viewed as less competent and less likable than a woman who dropped a less "offensive" but equally feminine item—a hair barrette—from her bag. The mere presence of the tampon also led participants to distance themselves physically from the woman, which suggests a disgust reaction, in which individuals avoid contact with contaminating entities. No wonder women heed the warnings of the advertisers! When others *find out*, indeed the consequences for women's social desirability are not favorable. The most interesting finding in this study was that the negative reaction to the tampon was generalized beyond the woman who dropped it to women in general. Participants reacted to the revelation of one woman's menstrual status by viewing women in general in a more objectified light. That is, they rated women's physical appearance as especially important relative to health and functioning in evaluating female bodies.

Why would hints about a woman's menstrual status lead to increased objectification of women in general? More generally, why would revelation of menstruation be a "problem" in the first place? Feminist theorists of the body (e.g., Martin, 1992; Rich, 1976) have argued that in patriarchal cultures, women's inferiority is defined by what separates them, or makes them different, from men. Because men hold the power to name, they define their own bodies and behavior as "normal" and "good," whereas features that differentiate women from men are viewed as "abnormal" and "bad," hence inferior. Women's reproductive systems are clearly different from men's. Consequently, the bodily functions associated with this system (e.g., menstruation, lactation, childbirth) become emblems of women's inferiority and the subjects of derogation. From this perspective, then, reminders of menstruation lead to reduced perceptions of competence, reduced liking, physical distancing, and increased objectification of women in general because they accentuate one important difference between women and men. Given the status difference inherent in patriarchy, accentuating this important biological difference between the genders leads to the negative association with women's characteristics. Consistent with this view, Gloria Steinem (1983) once admonished that if men (those with the power to name) menstruated, "it would become an enviable, boast-worthy, masculine event . . . men would brag about how long and how much" (p. 338).

WOMEN'S SELF-OBJECTIFICATION AS FLIGHT FROM THE CORPOREAL BODY

Contemporary stereotypes about women are paradoxical, because they contain both negative and seemingly positive judgments. As Glick and Fiske (1996) have shown, women are simultaneously perceived as less competent and valuable than men, but are also idealized in their roles as wives and mothers. Another way in which views of women are paradoxical is in terms of their bodies. On the one hand, women's reproductive functions and body functions are viewed with derision, but, on the other hand, their bodies are revered as cultural symbols of beauty and male desire.

We have argued that women's corporeal bodies, and especially the bodily functions associated with menstruation, have served historically as emblems of women's inferiority in patriarchal societies. The measures that women take to conceal and control menstruation, and hence their association with nature, might thus be argued to become their passage to civilization and social acceptance in cultures that elevate the mind over the body. Further, not only is menstruation concealed, but, at least in Western cultures, a "civilized" female body is defined by ideals of beauty. Women spend enormous amounts of time and money transforming their physical bodies into idealized bodies through a mind-boggling array of methods, from make-up and fashion to dieting and even cosmetic surgery (cf., Wolf, 1991).

Whereas women's chronic attention to their bodies' outward appearance has been viewed over the ages as "vanity," the feminist perspective of objectification theory argues that such habitual body monitoring is actually a survival strategy in a sexually objectifying culture. And we believe one reason for this is that the sexually objectified body can become a means for women to flee the biological–i.e., "inferior"–body. The practices of self-objectification, despite their negative consequences for women's subjective experience, can also bring rewards. Women who are "eye-catching" and deemed attractive receive a host of interpersonal and even economic positive outcomes. As Unger (1979) has argued, physical beauty can function as a kind of currency for women. For example, physical attractiveness correlates more highly with popularity and marriage opportunities for women than for men (e.g., Berscheid, Dion, Walster, & Walster, 1971; Margolin & White, 1987). So women themselves, therefore, often participate willingly in the cultural flight away from the corporeal body, engaging in a great variety of body-altering practices designed to transform the physical body into the idealized body (e.g., Tiggemann & Kenyon, 1998).

NEGATIVE CONSEQUENCES FOR WOMEN'S BODILY KNOWLEDGE AND SELF-ACCEPTANCE

Feminist writers have described the ways in which a sexist culture yields women who are alienated and distant from their own bodies, and a significant part of the feminist movement of the 1970s involved educational efforts to reconnect women with their physical selves (e.g., Lerner, 1993; Rich, 1979). From the perspective of objectification theory, we would argue that one significant path to this alienation is women's engagement in self-objectifying practices as a way of fleeing the culturally threatening, messy body. These practices carry negative consequences for women's own bodily self-knowledge and acceptance.

There is indeed empirical evidence that women are less attuned to internal physiological information (such as heart rate, stomach contractions, genital vasodilation) than men and make relatively less use of such bodily cues than men do in determining their subjective feeling states (see Roberts & Pennebaker, 1995, for a review of these studies). One possible path through which self-objectification practices might lead to this insensitivity is through the self-conscious body-monitoring that we have argued occupies women in a sexually objectifying culture. Because many women are vigilantly attuned to their bodies' outward appearance, they may have limited perceptual resources to attend to inner body experience.

Self-objectification practices may function, therefore, to reduce the knowledge base women have regarding their own inner experience. Roberts (2000) has recently found that self-objectification also predicts more negative attitudes toward the body's physicality. In that study, women who held a more self-objectified perspective on their own bodies also held more negative attitudes toward menstruation, one of the body's most "creaturely" functions. It was those measures of self-objectification that tap into the appearance-monitoring and surveillance practices theorized by objectification theory to be psychologically taxing that showed the strongest correlations with negative attitudes toward menstruation. The more women engaged in such self-objectifying practices, the more they endorsed extremely negative feelings about their menstrual periods, including disgust, contempt, embarrassment, and shame.

We have established that self-objectification operates on the *individual* level to distance women from their bodies, supplant the privileged access they might normally have to their body's inner experience with a "looking-glass" view, and increase their feelings of self-loathing toward such bodily functions as menstruation. In addition, on the *cultural* level, it might be argued that the norms of secrecy and concealment that surround menstruation and other reproductive functions, which women tend to obey willingly and even enforce, may serve the function of keeping women's real, corporeal bodies out of the public eye. This leaves the sanitized, deodorized, hairless, impossibly idealized images the media provide us with as the *only* women's bodies we encounter and accept.

DEVELOPMENTAL CONSIDERATIONS

Women's attitudes toward their bodies and their menstruation are different at different points in the life course. As Chrisler (1988) has shown, younger women have more negative attitudes toward their periods than do older women. Research on adolescents' responses to menstruation suggest that girls experience mixed feelings about menarche and develop increasingly negative attitudes toward menstruation over the first few post-menarcheal years (Koff & Rierdan, 1995; Koff, Rierdan, & Jacobson, 1981; Ruble & Brooks-Gunn, 1982). Recall as well that younger women view their bodies through a more self-objectifying lens than do older women, and those who are more self-objectifying report more shame, self-loathing, and disgust in relation to menstruation (Roberts, 2000).

From a cognitive developmental point of view, it is no surprise that self-objectification emerges at puberty. Self-objectification requires taking the perspective of the other in comparing one's body to an outside ideal. Although perspective-taking emerges in middle childhood (Higgins, 1991; Selman, 1980), the capacity to entertain multiple perspectives and evaluate the self in light of alternative possibilities does not emerge until adolescence (see Harter, 1999, for review). Advances in perspective-taking and multidimensional thinking serve the task of identity formation that is associated with adolescence, but they may also help to explain the high levels of self-objectification at this age. Adolescents self-objectify not only because the culture provides models for them to do so, but because they can. It could be argued that media constructions of beauty and marketing of menstrual products become available in a new way for adolescents who use these images as bases for evaluation of the adequacy of the self. The heightened insecurities and self-consciousness associated with normative adolescent comparison-making are further heightened by advertising depictions of menstruation as something to be concealed and contained (Simes & Berg, 2001).

MENARCHE, SELF-OBJECTIFICATION, AND DEPRESSION

De-selfing. Beginning with puberty and continuing across the life course, girls and women are twice as likely to experience depression as boys and men (Nolen-Hoeksema, 1990). Researchers have suggested that women's greater attention to relationships may be linked to this gender difference (Miller, 1991). Miller's (1987) early formulations suggested that women's socialization toward caretaking leads them to suppress the needs of the self in the service of others and that this de-selfing is implicated in depressive symptoms.

Gilligan and colleagues (e.g., Brown & Gilligan, 1992) have argued that it is precisely at the point that girls reach adolescence and begin to take on an adult female form that they begin to lose voice in the relational realm. They suggested that as girls don the mantle of womanhood, including cultural expectations about femininity, they shed the self-assertions, clarity, and willingness to confront others that characterizes the voices of middle childhood girls (Brown & Gilligan, 1992). In the interest of serving the needs of others, keeping the peace, or maintaining harmony, girls silence or suppress their own needs, wishes, and desires. Loss of voice and subsequent de-selfing in the service of relationships has been associated, in the clinical literature, with depression in both adolescents and adults (e.g., Jack & Dill, 1992; Miller, 1987). Further, for girls and women who define themselves predominately through the matrix of relationships, lack of support and lack of mutuality in significant relationships has contributed to loss of voice and depressive symptoms (Genero, Miller, Surrey, & Baldwin, 1992; Harter et al., 1997; Harter, Waters, Whitesell, & Kastelic, 1998). In Harter et al.'s work (1998), these outcomes were most pernicious among girls who embraced a feminine stereotype.

Gilligan described the loss of voice accompanying girls' entry into puberty as a form of dissociation from their own experience in pursuit of sustaining relationships. Loss of voice, then, reflects a flight into relationship—a monitoring of shifts in the relational field and adjustment of one's own behavior to accommodate—that is analogous to the body checking, correcting, and monitoring from the perspective of the other that we associate with self-objectification. Self-objectification theory would suggest that it is the *construal of the self as a commodity* for the other's use that contributes to this de-selfing and, ultimately, to depressive symptomatology. Thus, to be a "being for others" as Jean Baker Miller described it, whether in the psychological and caretaking sense or as the object of the others' gaze, is to lose track of one's self as initiator and to consign oneself to the role of being looked at or acted upon.

Disparity between the real and the ideal body. A wide discrepancy between the real self and the ideal self has been associated with depression and low self-esteem (Harter, 1999; Horney, 1945; James, 1892; Rogers & Dymond, 1954). Dating typically begins at 12 to 13 years old in the U.S. (Cauffman & Steinberg, 1996), which places it just at the point of menarche and right at the time when the disparity between an adolescent body and a supermodel ideal are likely to be most pronounced. Considering that the average model weighs 20 pounds less than she did two decades ago and yet the average woman weighs more now than she did in the 1980s, modern adolescent girls face an increasingly exacting standard for beauty, and only a minute fraction of these girls at puberty will match this ideal (Smolak, Levine, & Gralen, 1993).

Individuals construct a self-concept drawing from many domains, but perception of one's physical appearance is the strongest correlate of self-esteem at all ages, and the correlation is strongest during adolescence (Harter, 1999). Perhaps due to the double standard for beauty, girls experience more body dissatisfaction than do boys beginning in late childhood and early adolescence, and this has been suggested as a contributing factor in gender differences in depression that begin at this age. In one study, adolescents who rated physical appearance as highly important to their self-concept also reported the highest levels of depression (Harter, Waters, & Whitesell, 1997). From the point of view of objectification theory, girls who overvalue physical appearance are likely to engage in self-objectifying comparison against an external standard, and the shortfall between their real bodies and the media ideal contributes to depression.

MENARCHE, SELF-OBJECTIFICATION, AND EATING DISORDERS

The literature on pubertal timing suggests a complex relationship between menarche and disordered eating. Many researchers have emphasized that the normative weight gain and shifts in the ratio of body fat to muscle that accompanies menarche contribute to concerns about the body and to the vigilance girls express in the form of dieting or disordered eating (Striegel-Moore, Silberstein, & Rodin, 1986). This vigilance is particularly prevalent among early maturing girls (Brooks-Gunn, 1987; Graber, Brooks-Gunn, Paikoff, & Warren, 1994; Simons & Blyth, 1987) whose weight gain during early puberty tends to be a larger percentage of their total body weight (Attie & Brooks-Gunn, 1989). Little or no information is given to girls about normative increases in body fat relative to muscle just prior to the onset of puberty. Although girls are instructed about the reproductive role of menarche, what they want is more information about what they can expect to feel and why (Koff & Reirdan, 1995). What they also need, it appears, is a more complete description of pubertal onset, one that normalizes weight changes that accompany puberty. In the absence of explicit education, these weight changes in prepubertal girls are ubiquitously interpreted as "fat" that requires "dieting." The silence of educators, parents, and other responsible adults about these normative developmental changes creates a void that is easily filled by advertisers of products.

Cauffman and Steinberg (1996) observed that it was not menarche per se, but the confluence of its onset with dating and sexual exploration that predicts eating disorders in early puberty. The girls in their study who were actively involved in dating were more critical of their own bodies, more likely to be dieting, and more likely to be engaged in disordered eating. Although self-objectification was not measured in this study, it seems likely that preoccupation and dissatisfaction with the body were exacerbated in these girls by the experience of being the object of the "gaze" in dating situations. This begs the question of what is going on in these early dating relationships. It appears that girls may interpret or experience men's attention at this age through a self-objectifying lens. Martin (1996) showed that girls believe that breast development serves as a signal of sexual availability to men and boys, which illustrates many girls' recognition at puberty that they are seen and evaluated as bodies, not as selves. Earlier research on what men and women look for in a partner suggests that these young women may not be misguided in their interpretations. In a study by Stiles, Gibbons, and Schnellmann (1987) men placed attractiveness and sexiness as the top two criteria for an ideal woman, whereas women placed these third and sixth, respectively, in their criteria for an ideal man. In such a dating context, self-objectification may emerge as part of a strategy for success in garnering the attention of the other sex.

A related issue is that the increase in the ratio of fat to muscle happens only in girls at this age. Thus, whether they are self-objectifying (mapping to the supermodel ideal or to the male gaze) or mapping themselves against a male standard of normalcy (one that is more muscular and less fat), girls are likely to view their own bodies as failing the test, and thus they may be predisposed to experience self-loathing and disordered eating during the pubertal transition. This is particularly true if they are early maturers (Cauffman & Steinberg, 1996; Simons & Blyth, 1995).

FEMINIST TREATMENT SUGGESTIONS

A feminist approach to the treatment of disorders associated with self-objectification maintains that eating disorders and the types of depressive symptoms we have detailed result from girls' and women's attempts to bend and shape themselves and their bodies to a standard of female adulthood that is punishing, unrealistic, and, we would argue, ultimately unhealthy. We have highlighted the onset of menarche as one gateway into the body-checking and self-monitoring of self-objectification. However, to treat conditions associated with self-objectification requires acknowledging that these psychopathologies have their roots more in the culture than in the individual. Hence, a critique of cultural constructions of women and women's bodies is at the core of feminist therapeutic interventions.

THERAPEUTIC IMPLICATIONS OF SELF-OBJECTIFICATION

We have argued that the development of self-objectification rests on normative developmental accomplishments in perspective-taking and multidimensionality of thought, because individuals must first be able to imagine the other's perspective (the gaze) and then make comparisons between themselves and an ideal. Let us now return to the example provided in the beginning of this article of a young woman with bodily self-loathing rooted in self-objectification. One feature of feminist therapy with self-objectifying young women could involve problematizing the possibilities for beauty offered by the dominant culture. In work with early and mid-adolescents, the therapist might ask girls to perform an exercise in perspective-taking: to treat, as an object of *their* gaze, the media images and messages that contribute to body shame over natural bodily functions (viz., menarche). Asking girls to bring in magazine images and advertisements depicting feminine hygiene products and discussing the lack of information actually conveyed in these advertisements both annoys and surprises girls. For example, one 12-year-old premenarcheal girl asked the second author, "Why is it that *American Girl* magazine tells you all about how to use a jacket to cover an 'accident,' but doesn't explain how to actually use the tampon if you find one?" She argued that "girls and boys should learn about these things from the time they're in preschool so it's just normal when it happens." The irony in this comment, of course, is that it is "just normal." Why doesn't it feel that way to premenarcheal girls? And how could the 18-year-old in our opening example be so disgusted by this "normal" process that she wished to remove her reproductive organs entirely? This 12-year-old's statement reflects what Simes and Berg (2001) labeled the "heightening insecurities" function of advertisements for feminine "hygiene" products. A feminist therapeutic model should explicitly challenge that function, and provide a venue for girls to create alternative formulations of menarche and of menstruation.

We have argued that the construal of the self as an object of the others' gaze constitutes a form of de-selfing. Thus, one aspect of treatments for disorders associated with self-objectification would be to bring the authentic self into the equation as one is evaluating one's body. A feminist therapeutic intervention could incorporate cognitive behavioral tools to assist the client in articulating an "authentic voice." For example, a first step would include examining the automatic thoughts, or cultural mandates that support self-objectification and menstrual shame. This could be followed by challenging the assumptions that underlie these automatic thoughts (problematizing the cultural mandate) and then creating alternative formulations (uncovering an authentic voice). As Roberts (2000) has observed, higher self-objectification in women is associated with greater endorsement of statements such as "I am embarrassed when I have to purchase menstrual products," "I find menstrual blood disgusting," and "When I have my period, I do things to hide the fact that I'm menstruating." Asking clients to challenge their beliefs about menstruation and to consider alternative formulations either as individuals or in a group setting is a good way to dismantle and, ultimately, change these cultural assumptions.

REDEFINING BODY: A FEMALE STANDARD

An investigation of the assumptions that frame menstrual blood as "disgusting" or "loathsome" is possible among young women with the cognitive complexity to challenge dominant cultural values. It is less likely, however, among early post-menarcheal girls, who are more likely than their "on-time" or "late" peers to be the targets of objectification by older boys, who may be most susceptible to self-objectification, and who suffer more negative psychological outcomes such as eating disorders (Cauffman & Steinberg, 1996). How, then, can these young women experience menarche as a natural and welcome manifestation of female

adulthood? They would have to be enjoined to welcome *female* adulth
cally, rather than adulthood generally, which is defined by a male standai~.
Koutroulis (2001) argued that menstrual bleeding is a stigmatizing behavior in societies with a patriarchal, White male standard of normalcy. As such, obscuring
the difference may reduce the stigma. If girls and women are empowered not to
hide their menstrual status, if indeed they sported their menstrual status as naturally as they do heavy coats in winter and light outerwear in summer, would this
increase the stigma or reduce it? The results of the Roberts et al. (2002) tam-
pon-drop experiment suggest that it might increase stigma for the bold few who do
it, and may have real consequences for perceptions of competence and likability.
Thus, an intervention for the girls and women who bleed and feel shamed if it is
discovered, would need to be couched in an activist framework. Recent movements to celebrate menarche with parties for daughters appear to be one developing effort in this regard, although as yet there are no data to indicate whether such
celebrations do indeed help to reduce stigma and negative feelings in girls about
their periods. Consciousness-raising exercises in which women wear a red ribbon
to connote that they are menstruating might also be undertaken as an educa-
tional/activist effort. The immediate results of such "outing" exercises may not reduce stigma, but would at least reveal to the participants their own complicity in
maintaining the status quo. Broader educational efforts to reduce secrecy and ignorance about menstrual processes must be aimed not only at women and girls,
but also at boys and men, if stigma is to be reduced. Explicit education concerning
normative changes in weight and fat to muscle ratios in girls and boys is needed as
well to assist people to redefine normalcy during puberty.

We have argued that self-objectifying girls may be prone to depression and
eating disorders because increasingly exacting cultural standards for female
beauty heighten the gap between real and ideal physical selves and because
self-objectifying girls overvalue appearance in their construction of a self-concept.
Research on self-image disparities suggests that one prophylactic against low
self-esteem and depression is *discounting* domains where the disparity between
real and ideal is wide. Thus, one intervention would be to find alternatives to the
overvaluation of appearance in the broader definition of self. Discounting the importance of appearance among this age group will be especially challenging.
However, because self-objectifying girls are more likely to feel the sting of the
disparity between their real bodies and the cultural ideal, another pathway for intervention might be *alteration of the ideal* against which girls make comparisons.
Construction of an ideal that more closely conforms to the realities of menarcheal
girls' lives, for example, through the group creation of photo essays of different
same-aged girls, might be one strategy for narrowing the gap between the real and
ideal.

We have suggested that self-objectification necessitates a flight from the body
via the appearance-monitoring practices required to sustain the perspective of the
other. If self-objectification constitutes a form of dissociation, then treatment of
disorders that arise from self-objectification necessitates reconnecting the individ-

ual to bodily states and competencies. Thus, one therapeutic task becomes suggesting activities that promote embodiment. Prescriptions could range from introducing a walking regime, or possibly dance or sport involvement, to encouraging clients to participate in activities that bring attention to one's internal states (e.g., meditation, authentic movement). Research suggests that a core distinction between those who self-objectify and those who do not is that descriptions of self-objectifiers focus on the *appearance* of their bodies, whereas those who do not engage in self-objectification highlight their physical *competencies* in describing their bodies (Noll & Fredrickson, 1998). Thus, therapeutic practices that promote reconnection with inner states as well as those that encourage the individual to experience body competence and joy, over time, might prove more compelling than the detached posture of self-objectification. Such a therapeutic intervention might be thought of as a way of helping girls and women to become more "full of themselves!"

CONCLUSION

We have argued that sexual objectification of the female body is broadly internalized by young girls and women in our culture and that this may produce ambivalent attitudes and attributions toward normal female body and reproductive functions (viz., menarche and menstruation). We have suggested that for those women and girls who have internalized these cultural standards to such a degree that they objectify their own bodies, the experience of the menstruating body is viewed even more negatively, and is characterized by self-loathing, disgust, and flight or dissociation from their corporeal selves. We have further suggested links between these phenomena and the rise of depression and disordered eating during adolescence. We believe that feminist therapeutic interventions aimed at psychopathologies associated with self-objectification could be enlivened by creating venues for girls' and women's critique of cultural mandates about the management of female bodily functions, by activities that foster increased appreciation for one's inner bodily experience, as well as those that promote experiences of body competence over appearance. Our feminist vision is that such therapeutic practices would promote resilience in the face of idealized media imagery and provide a healthier, more realistic, and even joyful sense of adult female embodiment.

REFERENCES

Aristotle. (1984). Generation of animals. In J. Barnes (Ed.), and A. Platt (Trans.), *The complete works of Aristotle*. Princeton, NJ: Princeton University Press.

Attie, I., & Brooks-Gunn, J. (1989). Development of eating problems in adolescence: A longitudinal study. *Developmental Psychology, 25*, 70-79.

Bem, S. L. (1981). Gender schema theory: A cognitive account of sex typing. *Psychological Review, 88*, 354-364.

Berscheid, E., Dion, K., Walster, E., & Walster, G.W. (1971). Physical attractiveness and dating choice: A test of the matching hypothesis. *Journal of Experimental Social Psychology, 7*, 173-189.

Brooks-Gunn, J. (1987). Pubertal processes and girls' psychological adaptation. In R. M. Lerner & T. T. Foch (Eds.), *Biological-psychosocial interactions in early adolescence* (pp. 124-153). Hillsdale, NJ: Erlbaum.

Brown, L. M., & Gilligan, C. (1992). *Meeting at the crossroads: Women's psychology and girls' development.* Cambridge, MA: Harvard University Press.

Cauffman, E., & Steinberg, L. (1996). Interactive effects of menarcheal status and dating on dieting and disordered eating among adolescent girls. *Developmental Psychology, 32*, 631-635.

Chrisler, J. C. (1988). Age, gender role orientation, and attitudes toward menstruation. *Psychological Reports, 63*, 827-834.

Coutts, L. B., & Berg, D. H. (1993). The portrayal of the menstruating woman in menstrual product advertisements. *Health Care for Women International, 14*, 179-191.

de Beauvoir, S. (1952). *The second sex.* New York: Random House.

Delaney, J., Lupton, M. J., & Toth, E. (1988). *The curse: A cultural history of menstruation.* Urbana, IL: University of Illinois Press.

Fredrickson, B. L., & Roberts, T. (1997). Objectification theory: Toward understanding women's lived experiences and mental health risks. *Psychology of Women Quarterly, 21*, 173-206.

Fredrickson, B. L., Roberts, T., Noll, S. M., Quinn, D. M., & Twenge, J. M. (1998). That swimsuit becomes you: Sex differences in self-objectification, restrained eating, and math performance. *Journal of Personality and Social Psychology, 75*, 269-284.

Freud, S. (1918/1964). Femininity. In J. Strachey (Trans.), *Complete psychological works* (Vol. 22). London: Hogarth Press.

Genero, N. P., Miller, J. B., Surrey, J., & Baldwin, L. M. (1992). Measuring perceived mutuality in close relationships: Validation of the Mutual Psychological Development Questionnaire. *Journal of Family Psychology, 6*, 36-48.

Glick, P., & Fiske, S. T. (1996). The Ambivalent Sexism Inventory: Differentiating hostile and benevolent sexism. *Journal of Personality and Social Psychology, 70*, 491-512.

Graber, J., Brooks-Gunn, J., Paikoff, R., & Warren, M. (1994). Predictions of eating problems: An 8-year study of adolescent girls. *Developmental Psychology, 30*, 823-834.

Harter, S. (1999). *The construction of the self: A developmental perspective.* New York: Guilford Press.

Harter, S., Waters, P. L., Pettitt, L., Whitesell, N., Kofkin, J., & Jordan, J. V. (1997). Autonomy and connectedness as dimensions of relationship style in adult men and women. *Journal of Social and Personal Relationships, 14*, 147-164.

Harter, S., Waters, P. L., & Whitesell, N. (1997). False self behavior and lack of voice among adolescent males and females. *Educational Psychologist, 32*, 153-173.

Harter, S., Waters, P. L., Whitesell, N., & Kastelic, D. (1998). Predictors of level of voice among high school females and males: Relational context, support, and gender orientation. *Developmental Psychology, 34*, 1-10.

Havens, B. B., & Swenson, I. (1988). Imagery associated with menstruation in advertising targeted to adolescent women. *Adolescence, 23*, 89-97.

Higgins, E. T. (1991). Development of self-regulatory and self-evaluative processes: Costs, benefits, and tradeoffs. In M. R. Gunnar & L. A. Sroufe (Eds.), *Self processes and development: The Minnesota Symposia on Child Development* (Vol. 23, pp. 135-166). Hillsdale, NJ: Erlbaum.

Horney, K. (1945). *Our inner conflicts*. New York: Basic Books.

Jack, D. C., & Dill, D. (1992). The Silencing the Self Scale: Schemas of intimacy associated with depression. *Psychology of Women Quarterly, 16*, 97-106.

James, W. (1892). *Psychology: The briefer course*. New York: Henry Holt.

Kaschak, E. (1992). *Engendered lives: A new psychology of women's experience*. New York: Basic Books.

Kissling, E. A. (1996). "That's just a basic teen-age rule": Girls' linguistic strategies for managing the menstrual communication taboo. *Journal of Applied Communication Research, 24*, 292-309.

Koff, E., & Rierdan, J. (1995). Preparing girls for menstruation: Recommendations from adolescent girls. *Adolescence, 30*, 795-812.

Koff, E., Rierdan, J., & Jacobson, S. (1981). The personal and interpersonal significance of menarche. *Journal of the American Academy of Child Psychiatry, 20*, 148-158.

Koutroulis, G. (2001). Soiled identity: Memory work narratives of menstruation. *Health, 5*(2), 187-205.

Lee, J. (1994). Menarche and the (hetero)sexualization of the female body. *Gender & Society, 8*, 343-362.

Lerner, H. G. (1993). *The dance of deception: Pretending and truth-telling in women's lives*. New York: Harper Collins.

Margolin, L., & White, L. (1987). The continuing role of physical attractiveness in marriage. *Journal of Marriage and the Family, 49*, 21-27.

Martin, E. (1992). *The woman in the body: A cultural analysis of reproduction*. Boston, MA: Beacon Press.

Martin, K. (1996). *Puberty, sexuality, and the self: Boys and girls at adolescence*. New York: Routledge.

McKinley, N. M., & Hyde, J. S. (1996). The Objectified Body Consciousness Scale. *Psychology of Women Quarterly, 20*, 181-215.

Miller, J. (1987). *Toward a new psychology of women* (2nd ed.). Boston: Beacon Press.

Miller, J. (1991). The development of women's sense of self. In J. V. Jordan, A. C. Kaplan, J. B. Miller, I. P. Stiver, & J. L. Surrey (Eds.), *Women's growth in connection: Writings from the Stone Center*. New York: Guilford Press.

Nolen-Hoeksema, S. (1990). *Sex differences in depression*. Stanford, CA: Stanford University Press.

Noll, S. M., & Fredrickson, B. L. (1998). A mediational model linking self-objectification, body shame, disordered eating. *Psychology of Women Quarterly, 22*, 623-636.

Rich, A. (1976). *Of woman born*. New York: Bantam.

Roberts, T-A. (2000, March). *"Female trouble": Self-objectification and women's atti-tudes toward menstruation.* Paper presented at the annual meeting of the Association of Women in Psychology, Salt Lake City, UT.

Roberts, T-A., Gettman, J. Y., Konik, J., & Fredrickson, B. L. (2000, January). *"Mere expo-sure": Gender differences in the negative effects of priming a state of self-objectification.* Paper presented at the annual meeting of the Society for Personality and Social Psychol-ogy, San Antonio, TX.

Roberts, T-A., Goldenberg, J. L., Power, C., & Pyszczynski, T. (2002). "Feminine protec-tion": The effects of menstruation on attitudes toward women. *Psychology of Women Quarterly, 26,* 131-139.

Roberts, T-A., & Pennebaker, J. W. (1995). Gender differences in perceiving internal state: Toward a his and hers model of perceptual cue use. *Advance in Experimental Social Psychology 27,* 143-175.

Rogers, C., & Dymond, R. (1954). *Psychotherapy and personality change.* Chicago: Uni-versity of Chicago Press.

Ruble, D. N., & Brooks-Gunn, J. (1982). The experience of menarche. *Child Development, 53,* 1537-1566.

Selman, R. L. (1980). *The growth of interpersonal understanding.* New York: Academic Press.

Simes, M. R., & Berg, D. H. (2001). Surreptitious learning: Menarche and menstrual prod-uct advertisement. *Health Care for Women International, 22,* 455-469.

Simons, R. G., & Blyth, D. A. (1987). *Moving into adolescence: The impact of pubertal change and school context.* Hawthorne, NJ: Aldine.

Slonim, R. (1996). *Total immersion.* Northvale, NJ: Aronson.

Smolak, L., Levine, M. P., & Gralen, S. (1993). The impact of puberty and dating on eating problems among middle school girls. *Journal of Youth and Adolescence, 22,* 355-368.

Steinem, G. (1983). *Outrageous acts and everyday rebellions.* New York: Signet.

Stiles, D., Gibbons, J. L., & Schnellmann, J. (1987). Young adolescents' images of the ideal woman and man. *Journal of Early Adolescence, 7,* 411-427.

Striegel-Moore, R. H., Silberstein, L. R., & Rodin, J. (1986). Toward an understanding of risk factors for bulimia. *American Psychologist, 41,* 246-263.

Tampax Report, The. (1981). New York: Ruder, Finn, & Rotman.

Tauna, N. (1993). *The less noble sex: Scientific, religious, and philosophical conceptions of women's nature.* Indianapolis: Indiana University Press.

Tiggemann, M., & Kenyon, S. J. (1998). The hairlessness norm: The removal of body hair in women. *Sex Roles, 39,* 873-885.

Unger, R. K. (1979). *Female and male.* New York: Harper and Row.

Ussher, J. (1989). *The psychology of the female body.* New York: Routledge.

Whelan, E. M. (1975). Attitudes toward menstruation. *Studies in Family Planning, 6,* 106-108.

Wolf, N. (1991). *The beauty myth: How images of beauty are used against women.* New York: Morrow.

Young, I. M. (1990). *Throwing like a girl and other essays in feminist philosophy and so-cial theory.* Bloomington, IN: Indiana University Press.

Making Menarche Positive and Powerful for Both Mother and Daughter

Jessica B. Gillooly

SUMMARY. Psychotherapists who treat mothers with preadolescent daughters are in an excellent position to positively influence mother-daughter relationships at a time when Western societal influences are pushing them apart. Therapists are encouraged to help mothers process their own experiences with menarche, development of secondary sexual characteristics, and attitudes toward their bodies. By exploring these areas with their clients and then by encouraging the mothers to have early intimate discussions with their daughters, therapists can learn valuable information about their clients and can lay the groundwork for healthier mother-daughter relationships. Examples are given to help therapists encourage mothers to begin these difficult dialogues with their daughters. Suggestions are presented to help mothers overcome their daughters' reluctance to discuss sensitive topics of bodily maturation, menstruation, and emerging sexual development. *[Article copies available for a fee from The Haworth Document Delivery Service: 1-800-HAWORTH. E-mail address:*

Jessica B. Gillooly, MFT, PhD, is a California-licensed marriage and family therapist who continues her private practice of 23 years in the Los Angeles area. She is also Associate Professor of Psychology at Glendale Community College where she teaches courses on health psychology and the psychology of women.

Address correspondence to: Jessica B. Gillooly, PhD, Department of Psychology, Glendale Community College, 1500 N. Verdugo Rd., Glendale, CA 91208 (E-mail: gillooly@glendale.edu).

[Haworth co-indexing entry note]: "Making Menarche Positive and Powerful for Both Mother and Daughter." Gillooly, Jessica B. Co-published simultaneously in *Women & Therapy* (The Haworth Press, Inc.) Vol. 27, No. 3/4, 2004, pp. 23-35; and: *From Menarche to Menopause: The Female Body in Feminist Therapy* (ed: Joan C. Chrisler) The Haworth Press, Inc., 2004, pp. 23-35. Single or multiple copies of this article are available for a fee from The Haworth Document Delivery Service [1-800-HAWORTH, 9:00 a.m. - 5:00 p.m. (EST). E-mail address: docdelivery@haworthpress.com].

KEYWORDS. Menarche, menstruation, mother-daughter connectedness, adolescence

In our modern secular culture few personal rites of passage are treated as important public events. Menarche in particular has been overlooked as an important rite of passage and has most often been relegated to an unobserved and unspoken occurrence in a girl's life. Her menarche is known and shared only with her mother and a few intimate friends, when it is shared at all (Brooks-Gunn & Warren, 1989; Houppert, 1999). Therapists who are providing psychotherapy to mothers of preadolescent girls are in a unique position to impact the mother-daughter relationship positively over an extended period of time. Therapists can and should play an important role in ensuring that the mother has the self-knowledge and the tools necessary to guide her daughter through intimate, meaningful communications about secondary sex characteristic changes and menstruation long before they occur. These early intimate mother-daughter discussions about body changes and menstruation can lay the groundwork for continued connected conversations about the teenage pressures of dating, emerging sexuality, break-ups, drug use, STDs, and other topics vital to self-protection (Sieving, McNeely, & Blum, 2000).

How a mother relates to her daughter concerning the issues of menarche and menstruation can determine how intimate and open the daughter will be with her mother for years to come. Just as importantly, a young girl's attitude about her own body, an important component of her emerging self-image, can be powerfully influenced by the mother's willingness to share the menarche experience with her daughter. In the Kaiser Family Foundation and Children Now survey (1999), it was reported that children aged 10 to 12 wanted more information and guidance from their parents. The Kaiser Family Foundation named their report "Talking With Kids About Tough Issues." They concluded that children 10 to 12 years old look to their parents as their primary source of information, especially about the serious, sensitive issues of developing bodies, sexuality, and peer pressures. After my own interviews with and gathering personal accounts about waiting for and beginning menstruation from preadolescent and adolescent girls and after reading hundreds of personal stories written by women aged 17 to 64 from my Psychology of Women classes, one main theme emerged: young girls' fears and anxieties were relieved when their mothers talked with them about menstruation before it happened (Chrisler & Zittel, 1998; Gillooly, 1998; Koff & Rierdan, 1995; Whisnan & Zegans, 1975). Despite the importance of this shared mother-daughter experience, most mothers in Western cultures feel ill-prepared and awkward discussing menarche with their daughters, and most daughters initially resist hearing anything about the topic from their mothers (Gillooly, 1998). Yet this is an area where psychotherapists can assist mothers to begin these meaningful conversations with their daughters.

WHY ARE MOTHERS SO FEARFUL AND HESITANT ABOUT INITIATING INTIMATE DISCUSSIONS WITH THEIR DAUGHTERS ABOUT MENARCHE?

Unfortunately, many women regard the task of informing their daughters about menarche as necessary but difficult to initiate. The uniquely female bodily process we call menstruation is somewhat confusing to explain and to understand. It has its own unique vocabulary, both formal and vernacular, and its own mythology. Each semester in my college Psychology of Women classes, I am reminded of how complex the menstrual cycle process is to teach and comprehend. My women students are reluctant to ask me questions about their bodies because they do not want to appear uninformed. Yet many of them have wanted this knowledge for years. If women think that they are uninformed about the specifics of the menstrual cycle, then it will make it less likely that they will feel comfortable initiating conversations about menstruation with their daughters.

After more than twenty years of private practice as a family psychotherapist, I have heard women relate how their own mothers' inabilities to discuss menstruation and other related topics led them to feel self-conscious and awkward about their developing bodies. They wanted their mothers to feel comfortable talking with them. And in turn, my clients expressed a desire for their daughters to make the transition into menstruation with as little fear, shame, and embarrassment as possible. The mothers often recalled having experienced one or more of those negative feelings when they were younger. Some mothers remembered feeling ashamed because they didn't know all of the facts about menstruation when they were young, and they recalled getting teased about their ignorance by other girls (or boys). Many women remembered either their own embarrassing girlhood "accidents" during school or social occasions or those of other girls that filled them with the fear that accidents could happen to them. Most women confess to feeling anxiety associated with the possibility of starting their period at the "wrong" time, for example, during graduation or on their wedding day. With such negative memories, it is no wonder that many women avoid or postpone the topic with their daughters until after they have reached menarche.

CULTURAL ATTITUDES AND PREJUDICES

There are almost no published personal stories of menarche in the popular press or in novels, yet more than half of the adult population has such a story to tell (Chrisler & Zittel, 1998; Lee & Sasser-Coen, 1996). This silence has to do with the attitudes and behaviors toward menstruation that our society carries as cultural norms. Although individuals may have their own personal beliefs about appropriate behavior, mainstream middle class Americans share a sense of what is acceptable, important, embarrassing, or shameful in every area of human behavior, including menstruation (Kissling, 2002). There are many books available that skillfully deal with the issues of biology and hygiene and are written for a teenage reader. Pediatricians and school nurses are good sources of accurate information, but they are careful to stick only to those same two topics. They rightly have concerns about interfering with family and cultural values, and they trust that the parents are doing their job.

Advertisements for tampons and other sanitary supplies are now commonplace on television and in the print media. Advertisers treat menstruation exclusively as a hygiene issue to be masked with perfumed pads and other products (Houppert, 1999; Merskin, 1999; Simes & Berg, 2001). Young girls quickly pick up from the world around them that silence and secrecy are the watchwords when the topic of menstruation is raised. The challenge for the mother who is contemplating what information and attitudes toward menarche to convey to her daughter is to develop a meaningful, personal, and positive message. It is at this moment that the therapist can be best of service to his or her client.

MOTHER AS EXPERT

By the time most girls are aged 8 or 9 they have heard sensational stories filled with erroneous information about menstruation and girls' ability to become pregnant (Rierdan, Koff, & Flaherty, 1985). Young girls desperately crave accurate information, but aren't sure whom to trust. Perhaps they have heard something from a friend at school, an older sister, or possibly a lecture from a school nurse or someone else in authority about the hygiene issues of menstruation. If they have older sisters, they might have heard their sisters' firsthand stories about when they "got it." Whether she acknowledges it or not, a girl at this age wants to hear from her mother about this new and confusing subject. And she wants not just facts and explanations; she wants to hear her mother's stories about her own menstruation (Gillooly, 1998). She expects her mother to be an expert on the subject because her mother has lived with "it" all her adult life, and she has every right not to be disappointed.

The difficulty for most mothers in discussing menstruation with their daughters stems not from the descriptions of the physical changes that the daughter is about to undergo, but rather from the sexual and emotional aspects that accompany the physical changes (Ellis, McFadyen-Ketchum, Dodge, Pettot, & Bates, 1999). Menarche is a visible rite of passage for young girls, even if it is no longer celebrated as such in modern Western cultures. Today many mothers and daughters are beginning to have small celebrations of this rite of passage. Mothers who are open to sharing stories, disbursing information, and accepting fluctuating emotions provide the much needed assurance and reassurance that their daughters need about their upcoming experiences with menstruation and the information about its relationship to pregnancy (McNeely et al., 2002).

The therapist has an important role in convincing the mother that she truly is an expert in the story of her own menstruation. I am not referring here to the "science" of menstruation, although getting the facts straight and learning the correct terminology will help the mother feel more confident when she begins talking with her daughter. I am referring to the rich personal journey of self-discovery that begins for every young girl when she starts to menstruate. Girls are capable of getting the facts about menstruation from almost anyone. Only someone whom they are sure knows them and loves them can give them the meaning and relevance of this important event in their lives.

One very important activity that therapists can ask their clients who are mothers of daughters aged 8 to 12 to do is to write their own life stories about menstruation. This will help prepare the mothers for their talks with their daughters about menarche and also give valuable information to the therapists about their clients. After the mother and therapist have discussed the mother's memory of her menarche, the mother will have more clarity about her own life as well as more confidence in helping her daughter to grasp the meaning of her own menstrual story. Almost all women remember when they reached menarche, but some women find it difficult to write their personal stories because they have never thought that their memories concerning menstruation were very important. When researching women's life stories for her dissertation, psychotherapist Wanda Johnson (1984) found that most women did not include their menarche story as one of their life stories. When she questioned them, the women readily admitted that menstruation had played an important part in their lives. Yet it had not even occurred to them to talk about menstruation as a significant event.

Mothers must be encouraged to believe that their personal menstruation stories are significant both to them and to their daughters. Also, by "getting in touch" with past feelings and experiences, mothers will be more sensitive to what their daughters might be feeling. However, if the mother's experiences include severe menstrual cramping, difficulties with fertility, or surgery connected with her reproductive organs or if her childhood or sexual experiences involved sexual and/or physical abuse or severe illness, her memories will most probably be negative ones, and special care and attention from the therapist is in order to prepare the client to support her daughter.

Any one of these traumatic experiences has the potential for lifelong consequences that will deeply affect mothers' feelings about their sexuality. The mothers' negative feelings about menstruation may inadvertently be passed on to their daughters. During the eight semesters that I assigned my students in the undergraduate Psychology of Women course the task of writing their stories of learning about and experiencing menstruation, I was surprised to read how the daughters' understood and interpreted their mothers' view of menstruation. If the mothers communicated a positive view, then the daughters for the most part also presented a positive view of their menstruation. If the mothers presented a negative view, such as calling menstruation "The Curse" or other such names, the daughters were more likely to hold a similar view of menstruation. Consequently, I have asked my female clients to write their menstrual stories. When their experiences included trauma related to their menstrual cycle, then I worked with them to separate their menstrual cycle from the trauma. I have worked with women clients who began to menstruate immediately after being raped, or were raped during their menstrual flow. Often the disgust and anger at the rape is locked together with menstruation in the women's memory. Helping a woman to understand that these two events are not causal can help her to normalize her feelings for her healthy female bodily functions. Likewise, women who were embarrassed or made to feel ashamed about their developing bodies and/or menstruation can also present theirs and others' menstruation in a negative manner. Sometimes I find that even causal comments by their mothers or fathers about menstruation can influence the clients' opinion for years. When a psychotherapist works with women to accept menstruation as a normal, healthy bodily function, then the women have a chance to relate to their daughters' changing body with acceptance, also. Most mothers say that they want their daughters to have a positive experience with menstruation, therefore, they are ready to present a helpful view of menstruation for their daughters.

THINKING LIKE AN 8-YEAR-OLD

Mothers need to begin conversations about maturation, changing bodies, and menstruation when daughters are around 8 years old. Mothers almost always find it difficult to believe that they need to talk to their daughters at such a young age. Yet if the daughter is between 8 and 10 years of age, her body is already beginning to mature. A hormone from her pituitary gland is being released into her blood supply while she sleeps. In the United States, children have been growing larger and maturing earlier since the beginning of the 1900s. In the past 100 years, the average age of a girl's first menstrual cycle has decreased from approximately 14 years, 2 months to an average of 12 years. Currently girls as young as 9 years of age have begun their regular menstrual cycles. No one is absolutely certain why children are maturing younger.

Herman-Giddens and colleagues (1997) analyzed average ages at which 17,077 young girls in the United States experienced pubertal changes. They found that the average age for breast development was 8 years 8 months for African-American girls and 9 years 10 months for European American girls. In fact, breast development and/or pubic hair growth was found in 3 percent of African-American girls and 1 percent of European American girls at age 3 years. The most accepted theory for why girls are developing at younger ages is that improved health care has increased children's weight and growth rates. Children in the United States receive the benefits of prenatal and postnatal vitamins, enriched foods such as milk and bread, and overall improved nutrition and health care. Any or all of these can lead to increased body weight that is necessary to trigger the onset of adolescence.

Because young girls' cognitive abilities are still more concrete than conceptual, a common problem is confusion with their mothers' explanation of menstruation terms. "Eggs" are more likely to be thought of as something to be scrambled and eaten for breakfast than as ova stored in women's bodies; to "fertilize" something conjures images of grandpa spreading manure around the tomato plants rather than conception. There is a lot of complicated material for an 8-year-old girl to absorb and understand. This is especially true when menstruation and sexual intercourse are presented in the same discussion. Often mothers are talking about one thing, but their daughters are imagining something completely different. Therapists can help their clients to practice simple, easy explanations about menstruation to be tried with their daughters. This will also give the therapist the opportunity to make certain that the mothers are giving clear, accurate information to their daughters. Samples of explanations for young girls are given in my book (Gillooly, 1998).

DAUGHTERS RESIST LISTENING AND ASKING QUESTIONS

A mother may be ready to meet the challenge of teaching about menstruation only to find that her daughter is a reluctant learner. There are legitimate reasons why a daughter may resist communicating about menstruation. Some daughters are hesitant to talk about menstruation because it is a strange-sounding, unknown process and they feel self-conscious about their abilities to handle the new responsibilities and expectations. Occasionally a daughter will decide at the first hint of adolescent development that, because she does not want her body to change, it won't, regardless of information to the contrary. She may use magical thinking to excuse herself from learning about anything that she believes could not happen to her. She may be determined to control her own body and believe that she will never menstruate. Until a daughter is ready to let go of this thinking, she will be a most hesitant learner. Some girls even hang onto this myth of control until they actually start menstruating. A few women from my Psychology of Women course wrote in their personal stories that they were so determined not to mature and/or gain weight that they became anorexic as a way of avoiding it. Some exercised excessively or trained in athletics or dance as a means of resistance against menstruation. The therapist may want to pursue this thought if the client presents with evidence of eating disorders or excessive weight or diet concerns. In addition the therapist may want the mother to discuss her recollections of weight gain during adolescence and what she remembers about the ways family, peers, and others treated her. After exploring this information the therapist can then talk with the mother about positive ways to relate to her daughter's adolescent weight gain.

Another area of challenge is when mother-daughter dialogues about menstruation are not separated from dialogues about sexual activity. The emotionally loaded area of sex tends to overshadow the subject of menstruation, and both girls and their mothers can find themselves frustrated. The media are no help in this area. Films, TV, and music videos make sex graphic and visible, but menstruation remains invisible and silent. Popular culture urges girls to become possessions, sex objects, or observers rather than participants. Girls are being told that they are ugly without makeup, that thinner is better, and that they must always meet the expectations of others (especially men). In the midst of all of this bombardment, along comes mother trying to teach her daughter about one more way that she cannot control her body. Mothers should be prepared for the fact that initially all conversations with their young daughters will actually be more like a monologue in which the mother will be the only one talking (Gillooly, 1998). Developing new tactics to encourage daughter-mother dialogue prior to the first mother-daughter discussion will go a long way to making the process more successful. Here are a few activities that can help start conversations with young girls about menstruation.

1. Ask your clients to choose some short stories from Chapter One of Gillooly (1998) about young girls who are waiting for their periods and read them together. The mothers can then talk about their memories of waiting for their first period and ask their daughters what they are thinking or feeling.
2. Encourage your clients to check with the school to find out when their daughters will be studying menstruation, adolescence, and sexual development. Most teachers welcome questions and involvement from caring mothers. Once the mothers know what and when this material will be covered in school, then they can read the materials together, or read it separately. Either way the mothers can begin to reinforce the points that they think are most important.
3. Have your clients write their own stories of learning about and reaching menarche. Ask them to share their stories with you and then to share them with their daughters. Some editing may be involved because many women's menstrual experiences involve incest, rape, pain, shame, and embarrassment. Most mothers say that they want

their daughters to feel positive about their approaching menstruation and do not want to pass this kind of information to their young daughters. As therapists you will be able to help the mothers process their troubling memories and feelings about menstruation and to help them relate to their daughters' approaching menarche in a positive way.

4. Brainstorm with your clients all the places where girls could get their periods for the first time and what could be done. Then encourage the mothers to ask their daughters about all the places they might start their periods and practice problem solving together. If the mothers will share their experiences, it can bring laughter and a sense that the mothers and daughters are working as teams to solve problems that arise in young girls' lives.

If your clients say that their daughters are completely resistant to the above suggestions, then here are a few more ideas. The mothers of these daughters need to be encouraged not to give up, but to continue with the monologues because they will eventually lead to dialogues. Mothers can say something similar to these:

1. "I'm craving chocolate today. This usually means that I'm going to start my period in a day or two. I wonder how you'll know when you will start your period. What do you imagine?"

2. "When I was your age my mother was embarrassed to talk about menstruation. I don't feel embarrassed to talk with you about menstruation. Could it be that my mother's embarrassment skipped my generation and was passed directly to you? How do you think you are like your grandmother? Or different?"

3. "We're headed to the lake for the weekend. I think I had better pack some pads in case my period begins. Let's take a few pads that we have for you in case you start your period while we're there. Is there room in your luggage for your pads?"

4. "I bought a new book about menstruation. I'd like to show you the book and talk about it before you go to bed tonight. What time is best for you?"

The key is to encourage mothers in their continued efforts for dialogues with their daughters. Some daughters are very reluctant to talk about personal things. But, whether they know it or not, they still need to hear about their mothers' experiences and knowledge. Therapists can encourage the mothers to keep talking and sharing with their daughters. This can feel like a thankless, frustrating time for mothers, but daughters do open up with their thoughts and feelings. This is exactly what most mothers say they want with their daughters. And what daughters say they want with their mothers.

OUT OF THEIR CONTROL

As a girl's body and emotions change, she can feel "out of control," and she may take out her frustrations, confusion, and unexplained anger on those closest to her. Mothers often become the prime targets for their daughters' emotional outbursts and blame.

During adolescence a girl will gain weight and height, sprout pubic hair, grow breasts, have her first menstrual cycle, and may have a confusing array of emotions. These events all occur without the girl's consent all because of an increase in her circulating hormones. Many girls are embarrassed and scared about this lack of control. They believe that menstruation is nothing to be celebrated or proud of, especially because they did nothing to earn it and may not have even wanted it. Mothers need not relinquish all control or impose total control over their daughters' lives. They can help their daughters learn to exert some control over their physical well-being by encouraging them to exercise, to eat nutritious foods, to play sports, and to enjoy their friendships with other girls. These activities can help promote positive self-development and help give daughters the confidence that they can create healthy, fulfilling lives for themselves.

In our society, by early adolescence girls have learned to compare everything about themselves to their peers. They are aware of who plays key positions on their teams, who is the teacher's favorite, who always gets the lead in the drama productions, who is taller, who is prettier, and who is growing breasts. Social pressure on young girls to compare and evaluate themselves in relation to others is enormous (Eccles, Barber, Jozefowicz, Malenchuck, & Vida, 1999). This type of self-evaluation usually begins at around 7 or 8 years of age, and it is well ingrained by 12 years of age. Girls not only compare themselves to other girls and to boys their own age, but also to their older sisters, teachers, and mothers. Therefore, talking about the uniqueness of each individual helps daughters resist the temptation to believe in perfection and to strive for an impossible goal.

MOTHERS NEED TO PRACTICE ACCEPTANCE
AND TEACH SELF-ACCEPTANCE

In order to help her daughter learn self-acceptance, a mother must first accept herself as who she is. Mothers' "to do" lists can be endless. It is admirable to strive, achieve, and organize, but it is also important to remember that these activities do not define the person. The goal for mothers and daughters alike is to value themselves for their uniqueness.

Girls too soon grow critical of themselves. Recent studies have shown that many young girls thought that they were overweight and reported that they had dieted to lose weight (Flannery-Schroeder & Chrisler, 1996; Richards, Casper, &

Larson, 1990; Stein & Reichert, 1990; Stice, Presnell, & Bearman, 2001). Unfortunately, cultural messages are telling girls to be thin at the exact time that they are genetically programmed to gain weight. Estrogen, the hormone that is released at the beginning of puberty, affects the pelvis by changing its shape from a narrow, funnel-like structure to a broader, wider structure. The wider pelvis translates to the widening of the hips. This functional change is obviously vital for the natural birth of a normal weight baby. Therefore, this growth spurt not only allows a girl to reach her adult height, but also to mature her skeletal structure and female reproductive organs.

The goal for an emotionally healthy individual is to become accepting of one's own strengths and weaknesses, as well as the weaknesses and strengths of others. For some girls, this takes a long time. Therapists' waiting rooms are filled with adults still unable to accept themselves and others as they are. Mothers who can bring their own excitement, enthusiasm, and determination to teach their daughters about menstruation through the telling of their own personal stories increase the possibility that their daughters will have positive experiences associated with this extraordinary time of life. Just as important, these intimate early mother-daughter conversations lay the foundation for future discussions about developing sexuality, teenage pressures to use drugs, and other topics about which teenagers need their parents' insights to make wise decisions. If mothers and daughters have a sustained history of intimate, personal dialogues with each other, then the likelihood that they will continue to broach intimate subjects with each other is greatly increased (Blum, 2002).

Psychotherapists who have clients with preadolescent daughters can utilize their unique position to encourage the mothers to be proactive in their relationships with their daughters. By encouraging mothers to talk about their menstrual experiences, therapists have the opportunity to help their clients with any unresolved issues around their menstruation. After therapists have had ample time to work with their clients' attitudes toward menstruation, then an inquiry can be made about whether the mothers have talked with their daughters about menstruation. Therapists can then support their clients to begin or continue their conversations with their daughters by providing a safe environment for mothers to practice talks with their daughters and to debrief after their conversations. For mothers who are struggling with their own issues while mothering adolescent daughters, this can be a thankless, frustrating time. By supporting clients to continue talking and sharing with their daughters, therapists can make the difference necessary for mothers and daughters to have a meaningful relationship. This is exactly what most mothers say they want with their daughters and what most daughters say they want with their mothers. And therapists are in the unique position to facilitate connected mother-daughter relationships, especially those of clients and their adolescent daughters.

REFERENCES

Blum, R. W. (2002). *Mothers' influence on teen sex: Findings from the National Longitudinal Study of Adolescent Health.* Minneapolis, MN: University of Minnesota, Center for Adolescent Health and Development.

Brooks-Gunn, J., & Warren, M. (1989). Biological and social contributions to negative affect in young adolescent girls. *Child Development*, 60, 40-55.

Chrisler, J. C., & Zittel, C. B. (1998). Menarche stories: Reminiscences of college students from Lithuania, Malaysia, Sudan, and the United States. *Health Care for Women International*, 19, 303-313.

Eccles, J., Barber, B., Jozefowicz, D., Malenchuck, O., & Vida, M. (1999). Self evaluations of competence, task values and self esteem. In N. Johnson, M. Roberts, & J. Worell (Eds.), *Beyond appearance: A new look at adolescent girls.* Washington, DC: APA Books.

Ellis, B. J., McFadyen-Ketchum, S., Dodge, K. A., Pettot, G. S., & Bates, J. E. (1999). Quality of early family relationships and individual differences in the timing of pubertal maturation in girls: A longitudinal test of an evolutionary model. *Journal of Personality and Social Psychology*, 77, 387-401.

Flannery-Schroeder, E. C., & Chrisler, J. C. (1996). Body esteem, eating attitudes, and gender-role orientation in children. *Current Psychology*, 15, 235-248.

Gillooly, J. B. (1998). *Before she gets her period: Talking with your daughter about menstruation.* Los Angeles: Perspective Publishing.

Herman-Giddens, M., Slora, E. J., Wasserman, R. C., Bourdony, C. J., Bhapkat, M. V., Coch, G. G., & Hasemeier, C. M. (1997). Secondary sexual characteristics and menses in young girls seen in office practice: A study from the Pediatric Research in Office Settings Network. *Pediatrics*, 99, 501-512.

Houppert, K. (1999). *The curse: Confronting the last unmentionable taboo–menstruation.* New York: Farrar, Staus, & Giroux.

Kaiser Family Foundation and Children Now Report. (1999, March). *Talking with kids about tough issues.* Menlo Park, CA: Kaiser Family Foundation.

Kissling, E. A. (2002). On the rag on screen: Menarche in film and television. *Sex Roles*, 46, 5-12.

Koff, E., & Rierdan, J. (1995). Preparing girls for menstruation: Recommendations from adolescent girls. *Adolescence*, 30(120), 795-812.

Johnson, W. E. (1984). *Female life cycle development: An exploratory study with emphasis on adolescence.* Unpublished doctoral dissertation, United States International University, San Diego, CA.

Lee, J., & Sasser-Coen, J. (1996). *Blood stories: Menarche and the politics of the female body in contemporary U.S. Society.* New York: Routledge.

McNeely, C. A., Shew, M. L., Beuhring, T., Sieving, R., Miller, B. C., & Blum, R. W. (2002). Mother's influence on adolescents' sexual debut. *Journal of Adolescent Health*, 31, 256-265.

Merskin, D. (1999). What every girl should know: Adolescence, advertising and the menstrual taboo. In S. Mazzarella & N. Pecora (Eds.), *Growing up girls* (pp. 113-132). Peter Lang Publishers.

Richards, M. H., Casper, R. C., & Larson, R. (1990). Weight and eating concerns among pre- and young adolescent boys and girls. *Journal of Adolescent Health Care*, 11, 203-209.

Rierdan, J., Koff, E., & Flaherty, J. (1985). Conceptions and misconceptions of menstruation. *Women & Health*, 10(4), 33-45.

Sieving, R. E., McNeely, C. A., & Blum, R. W. (2000). Maternal expectations, mother-child connectedness and adolescent sexual debut. *Archives of Pediatric Adolescent Medicine*, 154, 809-816.

Simes, M. R., & Berg, D. H. (2001). Surreptitious learning: Menarche and menstrual product advertisements. *Health Care for Women International*, 22, 455-469.

Stein, D., & Reichert, P. (1990). Extreme dieting in early adolescence. *Journal of Early Adolescence*, 10, 108-121.

Stice, E., Presnell, K., & Bearman, S. K. (2001). Relation of early menarche to depression, eating disorders, substance abuse, and comorbid psychopathology among adolescent girls. *Developmental Psychology*, 37, 608-619.

Whisnant, L., & Zegans, L. (1975). A study of attitudes toward menarche in White middle-class American adolescent girls. *American Journal of Psychiatry*, 132, 809-814.

Negative Attitudes Toward Menstruation: Implications for Disconnection Within Girls and Between Women

Margaret L. Stubbs
Daryl Costos

SUMMARY. In this article, we draw from a body of research in the last 20 years, our own included, to suggest a framework for thinking about how attitudes toward and experience with menstruation contribute to girls' and women's notions of what it means to be female, to be a woman. Building on the current relational framing of psychotherapy, that a client's conception of herself is tied to her efforts to connect with others, we argue that negative attitudes toward menstruation can cause females to be "disconnected" from one another. Taking a life span perspective, we discuss how adolescent girls receive mixed messages about menstruation, how college women reflect negative attitudes about menstruation,

Margaret L. Stubbs is an independent scholar who is currently Research Associate at the University of Pittsburgh School of Nursing. She is studying the impact of acupuncture on hot flashes with Dr. Susan Cohen. Daryl Costos, a personality psychologist, is a lecturer in the Department of Psychology at Boston University where she teaches courses in psychology of women and research methods.

Address correspondence to: Margaret L. Stubbs, 1105 Heberton Street, Pittsburgh, PA 15206.

Portions of this paper were presented at the June 1999 meeting of the Society for Menstrual Cycle Research, Tucson, AZ.

[Haworth co-indexing entry note]: "Negative Attitudes Toward Menstruation: Implications for Disconnection Within Girls and Between Women." Stubbs, Margaret L., and Daryl Costos. Co-published simultaneously in *Women & Therapy* (The Haworth Press, Inc.) Vol. 27, No. 3/4, 2004, pp. 37-54; and: *From Menarche to Menopause: The Female Body in Feminist Therapy* (ed: Joan C. Chrisler) The Haworth Press, Inc., 2004, pp. 37-54. Single or multiple copies of this article are available for a fee from The Haworth Document Delivery Service [1-800-HAWORTH, 9:00 a.m. - 5:00 p.m. (EST). E-mail address: docdelivery@haworthpress.com].

and how adult women's differing experiences with menstruation can lead to disconnection *between* women. Specifically, we find that negative attitudes toward menstruation can result in mother-daughter disconnection and put women at odds with one another with regard to how to manage menstrual distress, PMS, and menopause. We suggest that a biopsychosocial exploration of menstruation in feminist therapy is warranted and that mental health professionals can benefit from using such a framework as they seek to understand the presenting difficulties of female clients. *[Article copies available for a fee from The Haworth Document Delivery Service: 1-800-HAWORTH. E-mail address: <docdelivery@haworthpress.com> Website: <http://www.HaworthPress.com> © 2004 by The Haworth Press, Inc. All rights reserved.]*

KEYWORDS. Menstruation, premenstrual syndrome, mother-daughter relationships, disconnections between women

Relational theorists (e.g., Miller & Stiver, 1997) have challenged the traditional assumption that "producing a self-sufficient individual is the goal of human development" and that "a great many psychological problems have their origins in the early mother-infant relationship, especially in the mother's failure to allow the child to become fully independent and self sufficient" (p. 2). Miller and Stiver (1997) and colleagues posited another focus for understanding psychological development. From working with and listening to their women clients, they came to understand that the imperatives to become independent, control emotional expression, and separate from others, ignore at best and pathologize at worst many aspects of women's experience. Moreover, they believe that this view of "healthy" human development obscures from our collective consideration "how connection, not separation, leads to strong healthy people" (p. 3) and how serious and repeated disconnection can lead to psychological problems.

Relational theorists have suggested that therapeutic interventions must include a mutually empathic relationship between the therapist and the client so that the client feels safe enough to explore what Miller and Stiver (1997) termed the central relational paradox. The paradox is that many people, especially females, deny parts of their own experience or create negative self-constructs to stay in connection with others. In the course of relational therapy, a client has the potential to identify and examine strategies she has crafted to confront the central relational paradox in her own life and reevaluate their usefulness. This process is a necessary step toward making changes that have the potential to ease current and future difficulties in interpersonal relating.

In this article, we discuss the impact of negative attitudes toward menstruation on developing notions of what it means to be female. We argue that throughout the life span females are largely "disconnected" from their menstrual cycles, and especially from exploring the social-psychological aspects of the menstrual cycle. To that extent, we suggest that a biopsychosocial exploration of menstruation in feminist therapy is warranted, particularly within the context of the current relational framing of psychotherapy, vis-à-vis a client's conception of herself as a woman or as a source of strength or challenge in her struggle to connect with others. In our discussion, we draw from our experience of over 20 years, first, as researchers who have each investigated social-psychological aspects of the menstrual cycle, and second, as professors who have taught undergraduates about menstruation in courses on the psychology of women, women's health, and sexuality, in a variety of post-secondary institutions.

WHAT HAPPENS TO GIRLS DURING THE TRANSITION TO ADOLESCENCE: MIXED MESSAGES ABOUT MENSTRUATION SET THE STAGE FOR DISCONNECTION

Discussions of girls' development during pre- and early adolescence usually begin with details about the biological aspects of girls' pubertal development. Menarche, or first menstruation, is generally identified as a biological marker for maturity. Beginning to menstruate is a physical event that takes place toward the end of puberty, after many other pubertal events (e.g., height spurt, breast bud development, development of secondary sex characteristics) have already occurred.

In these descriptions of development, there is usually an acknowledgement that pubertal growth is accompanied by shifts in self-perception (e.g., Crawford & Unger, 2000). A reorganizing effect of puberty on girls' identity has been mentioned in the psychoanalytic literature (e.g., Kestenberg, 1967), and more recent data suggest that puberty focuses children's attention on the changing body and on the mature female body (Greene & Adams-Price, 1990). With respect to the impact of menarche on this refocusing, studies by Koff, Rierdan and their colleagues indicate that after menarche, there is an increase in identification with mature femininity; girls regard menstruation as a transformative experience that changes girls to more mature young women (Koff, 1983; Koff, Rierdan, & Silverstone, 1978; Rierdan & Koff, 1980).

The transformation is not, however, straightforwardly positive. Instead, identification with mature femininity is quite complex, in part because our culture is ambivalent about the value and meaning of the mature female body (Crawford & Unger, 2000). In addition, at the same time that girls are becoming more mature physically, they are also becoming more keenly observant and cognitively more capable of recognizing and grasping the particulars of the power relations in our society: girls come to understand that men are valued over women, and with this recognition they must decide how to deal with their lack of power as females (Brown & Gilligan, 1992).

Debold, Wilson, and Malave (1993) mentioned a few possible outcomes of what can happen during the transition to adolescence when girls are facing and trying to reconcile body image and gender-related power issues. Girls may follow a traditional path of feminine identity and give up parts of themselves in order to fit in with gender role norms within a patriarchal society. Another possible strategy is to devalue feminine identity altogether and strive to become "one of the guys." Or, a girl may seek to "have it all" by striving for traditional femininity at home and masculinity at work. As Debold et al. (1993) indicated, these paths are not only at odds with one another but they all require a girl to give up parts of herself.

As a physical, psychological, and symbolic maturational event, menarche carries mixed messages for girls about what it means to be female. Educational materials about menstruation congratulate girls on becoming women (one of the only positive aspects about menstruation to be mentioned) but at the same time emphasize that menstruation is a hygiene challenge during which girls should keep clean and be discrete (e.g., use products with the best absorbency, the slimmest pads, products that are easy to conceal and dispose of) so that no one will know when they are menstruating (Erchull, Chrisler, Gorman, & Johnston-Robledo, 2002; Houppert, 1999; Whisnant, Brett, & Zegans, 1975).

It is interesting that girls' attitudes reflect these mixed messages. Girls do acknowledge menstruation as a natural, normative event that signifies that they are growing up; they also worry about it, especially premenarcheal girls (Stubbs, Rierdan, & Koff, 1989), and some regard menstrual blood as disgusting or gross (Houppert, 1999; Williams, 1983). In addition, Lee and Sasser-Coen (1996) have reported how some girls describe being disconnected from their periods. Some girls talk about their periods as something that comes in from out of nowhere and just happens to them: "It's" an alien encounter; you "have or get" it, like the flu. It is reasonable to assume that the proscription to hide menstruation (either directly stated or more subtly conveyed in product advertisements that stress convenience) as a prominent message at the very beginning of girls' experience with menstruation sets the stage for women's psychological disconnection from menstruation.

WHAT COLLEGE STUDENTS THINK: DISCONNECTION CONTINUED

The college-aged students we work with evidence similar disconnection from menstruation.[1] Their disconnection emerges first in their resistance to studying the menstrual cycle in our courses, even when that course is the Psychology of Women. For example, Stubbs' students balk at seeing menstruation on the syllabus:

> . . . when I saw menstruation on the syllabus . . . I wondered what there was to learn on the subject. I had been through health and sex ed in high school and have been menstruating for roughly eight years. I figured I knew all I needed to know on the subject and time would have been better spent on something else . . . I had never thought about menstruation. It was just something, not horrific, but definitely inconvenient, that happened each month. If I was lucky, I got to skip a month. It was a little embarrassing, especially when I first started, but after eight years, I was getting over it. It just happened. It was part of being a woman . . . something bad that comes along with being a woman.

Stubbs' students are genuinely baffled by an assignment that asks them to identify and discuss with the class some positive aspect of the cycle. One student explained:

> I thought that an answer could not exist . . . I had never viewed my menstrual cycle as a healthy part of living, just something I had to endure if I wanted to have children someday . . . women today have nothing positive to report about their cycles.

Costos has experienced comparable resistance in her students. She requires students to conduct an in-depth interview about menstruation with a woman over 30 years of age and write a paper analyzing the interview in relation to course readings. She has found that many students are apprehensive about interviewing women about the topic of menstruation. Often their anxiety is only heightened when they begin to talk to others outside the class about the task. One student reported:

> "They want you to do *what*?" my roommate gasped.
> "What kind of class has you do *that*?" my aunt retorted.
> "How are you going to get 15 pages out of *that*?" my boss asked incredulously.
> "I'll make it easy for you: Eew, eew, eew, eew. Gross, gross, gross!" joked my best friend's mother.

Costos has discovered that many students are bewildered as to whether they know anyone who would agree to such an interview. "Can I interview my mother?" is a regular question in response to the assignment. Some students resolve the dilemma of whom to interview by choosing their mothers; they often explain that they have never before talked about the topic with their mothers. Thus, although uncertain about breaking the silence even with their mothers, many choose to do so because this seems "safer" than interviewing a stranger. Others are genuinely stymied by the task of finding an appropriate interviewee. Each semester at least one "desperate" class member is kindly aided by another classmate and introduced to "a woman who is willing to be interviewed about her period."

In addition to their initial resistance, our students are particularly negative about the cycle. Through her years of teaching, Stubbs has informally tracked her undergraduate students' knowledge about and attitudes toward menstruation. As a regular class exercise she surveys her students before their class sessions on menstruation and menarche, PMS, and menopause. Students then work in small groups to make tallies of the data and to compare their current attitudes and knowledge to information from required readings. Students are typically not able to describe what menstruation is or to name the four major hormones involved and how they fluctuate; they are confused about when ovulation happens (and what it actually is), and they do not differentiate between premenstrual and menstrual discomfort. Asked to name changes associated with menstruation, ovulation, and menopause, they list negative symptoms to the exclusion of positive or even neutral changes. Stubbs been getting the same results for over 10 years (Stubbs, Palmer, & Yandrich, 1999), and they match what she's found in more formal investigations of college student's attitudes toward menstruation.

For example, in one study women students from a private, urban college were asked to describe the physical, emotional, and intellectual changes associated with menstruation, ovulation, and menopause (Koff, Rierdan, & Stubbs, 1990). Participants responded with an overwhelming number of negative changes as compared with positive or neutral changes. In addition, these college-aged women did not know much more about menstrual cycle facts than junior high/middle school students did (Koff & Rierdan, 1995). Finally, the confusion that college-aged women evidenced with respect to knowing exactly what ovulation was and when it occurred is especially alarming, given that most college-aged people are sexually active. Stubbs replicated this study with college-aged women (and men) from a rural New England state university a few years later (Stubbs, 1993), and the findings were nearly identical.

Thus, both our formal data and classroom discussions indicate that college-aged women see menstruation as a negative aspect of being female. According to the young women we've worked with, the best time to be female is before age 10; after the beginning of menses, it's all downhill until, and even beyond, menopause. They conceived of menopause as "the rest of a woman's life," a time after menstrual periods cease that is characterized by fuzzy thinking, a lessening of intellectual capacity, depression, irritability, and a general, ever-degrading malaise, until death. This is hardly an inspiring view of what lies ahead for women!

In truth, what lies ahead is a life span of exposure to negativity about menstruation. Consider the following. At menarche, a girl is likely to have learned to be embarrassed by the subject. She may have gotten negative messages from school, her mother, her sisters, friends, or educational materials about menstruation (Costos, Ackerman, & Paradis, 2002; Lee & Sasser-Coen, 1996). She has learned that menstruation was not something to talk about especially with boys or fathers (Lee & Sasser-Coen, 1996). Thus, she has learned that menstruation is essentially a taboo topic even in these modern times. Menstrual product advertising has encouraged her to hide her menstruation from others, and in response, as she matures, she finds that she spends an annoying amount of time tending to menstrual management (surreptitiously carrying, storing, using, and discarding menstrual products). She may experience menstrual cramps and/or premenstrual syndrome (PMS) and/or know women who do. That being the case, she is likely to come to see the monthly time as a negative occurrence for her or others. Alternatively, she may experience symptom-free menstruation and feel at odds within a culture in which menstruation is assumed to be problematic. Throughout her lifetime, she hears nothing but put-downs in the media about PMS or advertisements for products to "treat" PMS (Chrisler & Levy, 1990; Erchull et al., 2002). The menstruating woman today has likely also heard from some quarters of the biomedical establishment that menstruation is obsolete (e.g., Coutinho & Segal, 1999) and, worse, is so hazardous to women's health that some researchers are trying to create a way to eliminate periods (hormonally) altogether. Told as a younger woman that she'd be healthier if she didn't menstruate, a woman approaching menopause learns that she would be healthier if she were to take hormones to combat the effects of "not having a period." She's advised that with the absence of regular periods, she may suffer from debilitating hot flashes, osteoporosis, heart disease, or mental decline. She is told that she may be emotionally distressed because she is "no longer a woman" (because she is no longer menstruating). And she is encouraged to consider hormone replacement therapy (HRT) to remediate both short- and long-term assumed menstrual-related afflictions.[2] It is, however, possible for her to have a baby postmenopausally, or serve as her infertile daughter's surrogate mother. The new reproductive technologies imply the ultimate irrelevance of the cycle, disconnecting it even further from women accustomed to acknowledging its traditional role in conception and childbearing.

THE CYCLE AS A SOURCE OF DISCONNECTION BETWEEN FEMALES

The menstrual cycle as currently interpreted in our culture can also lead to disconnections between women. We turn now to a discussion of these.

Mother-Daughter Disconnection

As mentioned earlier, girls at adolescence realize that men are valued over women in our society. Debold et al. (1993) argued that this discovery might lead to a disconnection between the mother and daughter as the daughter deals with the reality that because of their gender, she and her mother lack power. If the mother restricts her own and her daughter's behavior to traditional gender roles, the daughter may resist and feel betrayed by her mother.

Costos et al. (2002) have demonstrated that the messages that daughters receive about menstruation from their mothers are predominantly negative. In particular, one of the messages that some mothers give to their daughters about menstruation in an effort to help daughters assume a proper feminine gender role is that the daughters must "grin and bear" any discomfort that comes with menstruation. In other words, the message is that the right way to deal with menstruation is to keep quiet about it; the wrong way is to express discomfort and talk about it. One outcome of such a message is that women may be divided from one another into two camps: women who "grin and bear" it, and women who do not. As a result, mothers and daughters, as well as women in general, may find themselves alienated from one another because they find themselves on opposing sides as to whether one can or should "grin and bear" menstruation.

Costos et al. (2002) explained that because of the taboo associated with the topic of menstruation, very little has been done to address better communication between mothers and daughters and negative messages about menstruation have passed from one generation to the next. In order for things to change, we need to promote more constructive talk between mothers and daughters. On the one hand, we need to encourage mothers to understand the extent to which negative messages exist in our society about menstruation and the impact that these messages can have on their daughters' psychological experience at puberty and beyond. On the other hand, we need to help mothers map the way to a positive menstrual experience for their daughters (Gillooly, this volume; Stubbs, 1990).

Women's Different Experiences Lead to Disconnection

To suffer or not to suffer. Cycle variability and management challenges put women in opposition to other women. Women choose sides when it comes to how they view and manage their experience with menstruation. When they choose sides, they inevitably find they are at odds with other women. For simplicity's sake, one could argue that there are two groups of women: the sufferers and the nonsufferers. These two groups are disconnected from one another because they really don't understand one another's experience. The sufferers find their lives disrupted by the experience of menstruation, whereas the nonsufferers do not. The sufferers, who are already silenced by society due to the taboo nature of the topic, have to be careful about how much they talk about their experience lest they be judged negatively (e.g., sufferers are exaggerating; they just can't take it; it's all in their heads). Also divisive is the corollary belief that if a woman has the proper attitude, her problems with menstruation would go away. A woman should "grin and bear it" or see her period as something "normal and natural" and "get a grip." Once she has the right attitude, if she still has problems, it could be a result of her diet or lack of exercise, widely believed to cause problems with menstruation although there is little scientific evidence to support the notion. Ultimately, however, it's a woman's responsibility to "get herself under control," and clearly, if she has a real problem, she should see a *doctor*. Alternatively, nonsufferers may be seen as oddities (other than "real" women) in a culture that assumes that all women suffer or are incapacitated premenstrually and/or during menstruation. Or, women who do not experience menstrual-related symptoms may simply be thought of as "in denial."

PMS divides women. Costos (1995) has studied the different attitudes that women hold about PMS, and has argued that PMS serves as an arena in which the conflicts dividing women in our society are played out. In her model, attitudes toward PMS are depicted on a continuum that ranges from anti-feminist to pro-feminist. A person with an anti-feminist attitude may deny the existence of PMS or express hostility toward women who claim to have PMS, whereas a pro-feminist person seems aware of some of the social psychological ramifications of PMS and expresses concern about the ways in which PMS might be used to undermine women. Kruger and Costos (1997) examined attitudes toward PMS in a sample of adult women and found that 50% had a mildly pro-feminist attitude toward women with PMS, and 40% had a negative or ambivalent attitude toward women with PMS. Very few women reflected an awareness of the degree to which PMS might be dividing women from one another.

As an example of how the varying perspectives on PMS can be divisive, consider the popular statement regarding PMS: "She's just using it as an excuse." This particular phrase is widely used, reflects disapproval for the woman who has "used her PMS," and has a number of interpretations. One interpretation is: "It bothers me that she can't behave like women are supposed to," which essentially denies the woman's suffering in favor of allegiance to the gender role proscription to grin and bear it. A second meaning is: "She's just bringing things down for all women by complaining about her PMS," which also denies suffering because the woman is not being a team player. Another interpretation is: "No, really, she *is* just using it as an excuse," which suggests a woman who does not experience PMS says she does in order to get out of something she does not want to do. This behavior can aggravate other women who do not want to use a "gender card" to advantage.

Finally, Martin's (1987) work also illustrates how PMS leads to disconnections between women when she describes how PMS puts women in a double bind. On the one hand, if women accept the idea that women's performance is affected premenstrually, then they face discrimination because women are seen as less reliable and not as productive as men. On the other hand, if women do not acknowledge that women undergo premenstrual changes, then they abandon those women whose experience is unpleasant.

The menopausal divide. With respect to menopause, one issue that has been highly debated in the media and among women is the question of whether or not to use hormone replacement therapy (HRT) to medicate menopausal experience. Martellock and Costos (1997) found that with regard to willingness to take hormones, their participants were divided; approximately half of the women said that they were willing to use HRT and half said that they were unwilling and unsure. Younger women (ages 26-39) were more likely to say they were willing to take hormones, whereas the older women (ages 50-68) were more likely to resist the idea of taking hormones. Although there are a number of possible explanations for the differences between the age groups, the authors pointed to the contrasting experiences the two cohorts have had with hormones. The older group, the first generation to take the early oral contraceptives, later deemed unsafe, was skeptical, whereas the younger group, using today's oral contraceptives and trusting them to be safe, was comfortable with the use of hormones. Thus, part of the divisiveness around HRT may be a direct reflection of whether to trust a medical model or not. As a function of this debate, those who choose to take HRT may be judged as overly concerned with staying young, dependent on the patriarchal medical establishment, and victims of the pharmaceutical companies' sales pitches. Those who choose not to take HRT may be judged as "letting themselves go" and as foolish not to take advantage of technological advances. It will be interesting to follow this debate closely in the context of new data that casts doubt on HRT's assumed positive impact on older women's health (Writing Group for the Women's Health Initiative Investigators, 2002). We suggest that women's reactions to this news will reflect the same possibilities for connection/disconnection as they reconcile whether to continue or begin hormone treatment during this phase of life.

Given that girls' and women's attitudes toward and experiences with menstruation vary over the life course (Stubbs, 1985), we think it is reasonable to assume that attitudes and experiences also vary along with other factors, for example, sexual orientation or fertility status. The meaning of menstruation as a marker of femininity is likely quite different to lesbians who hold a variety of perspectives on whether and how to become mothers; similarly one's attitudes toward and experiences with the menstrual cycle are apt to be different for women who are trying to get pregnant and can't, than for women who are trying not to get pregnant but can.

In addition, actor-observer differences may play a role. Research indicates that men believe menstruation is more debilitating than women believe it is (e.g., Brooks-Gunn & Ruble, 1977; Chrisler, 1988; Parlee, 1974). These results raise the question of whether people who don't experience menstruation are more inclined to think of it as debilitating than are people who do experience it. Maybe menstruation is worse in the imagination than it is in reality. If actor-observer differences contribute to men's perceptions of the cycle, they may also have a role for women who are processing information about women who have different sorts of menstrual experience than they do.

We suggest that comparisons of different attitudes toward and experience with menstruation are likely to lead to disconnection given the current cultural context in which the totality of menstrual experience is so negatively regarded. A more inclusive, connected perspective requires a more complete examination of the biopsychosocial meaning of the cycle in women's lives than has been the case to date. It is to this discussion that we now turn.

MENSTRUAL EXPERIENCE AS SEEN THROUGH A BIOMEDICAL LENS

In order to understand the depth and persistence of negative views associated with the menstrual cycle, we suggest an analysis of our culture's interpretation of menstruation as primarily (essentially) a biological event. We believe that a deep-seated belief in the menstrual cycle as an essentially biological event is a bias that prevents us from seriously considering its social-psychological aspects. Most people have been led by our culture to believe that biology is primary. Even though they may have awareness of the nature-nurture controversy, most people tend to forget that there is an interaction between biology and environment. Even if they recognize such an interaction, many come down on the side of nature when trying to explain a physiological phenomenon because biological science is valued so highly in our culture. For example, though many people might be willing to say that stress might be a predictor of a behavior or a disease, they usually accept the idea that a pill will fix things.

The belief in biology as primary is especially evident when it comes to the topic of menstruation. Take, for example, the impact of menstrual-related products on the pharmaceutical industry. Premarin (estrogen for menopausal women) has been a best-selling drug. Egan (1985) was among the first to point out that overtrust of the medical model leads us in the direction of such questionable medications for PMS as progesterone. Recently this view has brought American women to accept the use of Prozac for the treatment of PMS, marketed under the name of Sarafem as a ploy to get around patent laws (Caplan, 2001). Feminist authors (Caplan, 2001; Chrisler, 1996; Egan, 1985; Lee & Sasser-Coen, 1996) who have written about the problem of reliance on the medical model are concerned that women are naïve about the social-psychological and political components of the experience of menstruation. It benefits the medical profession and the pharmaceutical industries to keep menstruation within the medical model. To do so represents the continued medicalization of women's experience, which has not always proved to enhance women's health, as feminist researchers have pointed out over the years (e.g., Gannon, 1998; MacPherson, 1981; Nash & Chrisler, 1997).

Against this backdrop, it is difficult to understand the social-psychological side of menstruation. When we talk about the psychological side of menstruation, essentially we are talking about how a woman's experience with menstruation may be influenced by her own or others' attitudes toward menstruation. There is evidence to suggest that negative views about menstruation in our society interact with a woman's experience. For example, in a classic study, Ruble (1977) was able to manipulate some of her participants into believing that they were premenstrual when they were not. Those who believed that they were premenstrual reported that they were currently experiencing more negative symptoms than a control group of women who had no expectations about the date of their next menstruation. In fact, all of the participants in the study were expecting their next periods in six or seven days, according to a questionnaire they completed before the testing session. The mere suggestion of premenstrual status elicited negative symptomatology from women.

Other important work on the impact of beliefs on experience was done by Golub (1976) and Sommer (1972). In those studies, although women reported negative moods premenstrually and during menstruation, and, moreover, believed that their performance on cognitive tasks would be negatively affected by menstruation, objective measures of performance failed to detect any performance decrements associated with the menstrual cycle. Their data reveal a firmly entrenched belief about menstruation held by many, even in the face of evidence to the contrary, that women are less capable during the menstrual and premenstrual phases of their cycles.

Feminist authors (e.g., Chrisler, 1996; Martin, 1987; Steinem, 1983) have addressed social-psychological issues related to menstruation and suggested that replacing our negative attitudes toward menstruation with positive ones could alter the experience significantly. Chrisler (1996) suggested that women should try to reinterpret their premenstrual changes in a positive way, which might lead to a much more positive experience. For example, one could reinterpret premenstrual tears as an adaptive way to cope with water retention instead of a signal of depression (Koeske, 1980).

Steinem (1983) also wrote about how an attitude shift would change the whole menstrual experience when she suggested that if men could menstruate, menstruation would be a celebratory event with noteworthy status. For example, men would brag about how long and how much they bleed. Critical to Steinem's point is that the status of women as the gender with less power leads to a negative attitude toward menstruation because it's something that only women do. In contrast, because men are the gender with more power, whatever they do is perceived in a positive way. If girls were congratulated for having reached menarche and given special treatment the experience of menstruation might be very different. Although accounts of cultural celebrations of menarche do exist (e.g., Delaney, Lupton, & Toth, 1988), there is no reason to assume that more elaborate positive rituals to mark this rite of passage for girls will emerge in Western culture, given the current trends to control the cycle (e.g., Coutinho & Segal, 1999) via hormonal treatment (to make it more predictable, less obtrusive or a supposed adjunct to enhanced health) or to manage the cycle's interruptions of both personal and work-related routines. Martin (1987) has also imagined the possibilities for a positive reinterpretation of the negative impact menstruation is thought to have on work performance. Women workers she interviewed did report a premenstrual decrease in work discipline (i.e., ability to maintain focus on work). Rather than seeing this behavior as problematic, Martin interpreted these findings as suggesting that women are less *willing* to tolerate work discipline premenstrually, although not necessarily less *able* to concentrate.

Martin (1987) argued that the expectation that people should perform consistently is a flaw in industrial societies. She pointed to other cultures that treat menstruation as a special time for women, and suggested that the premenstrual phase may be a time of heightened power and capacity for women for a different kind of concentration, a concentration that permits expression of one's innermost depths. What if menstruation was seen as a good thing and women were encouraged to take the day off if they desired to explore their enhanced sensitivities?

Martin (1987) also discussed premenstrual anger as one of the symptoms of PMS that is perceived by women as a sign that they are "not themselves." She suggested that women who have been socialized to meet gender role expectations by being happy and helpful might be most distressed by their feelings of anger. However, even anger may be seen in a constructive way. Martin believes that premenstrual anger may be symbolic of a woman's monthly reminder of her secondary status in society; thus, it should be embraced as legitimate. She and other feminist researchers who address this issue (e.g., Chrisler & Caplan, 2002; Chrisler & Johnston-Robledo, 2002) would suggest that feminist therapists encourage women to use their premenstrual anger to fight oppression.

IMPLICATIONS FOR THERAPY

One goal of feminist therapy is to help clients see the social context in which their psychological difficulties are occurring (Crawford & Unger, 2000). We believe that the sociocultural context in which women experience menstruation is not well understood either by the general public, including most women, or by mental health practitioners. In order for most people to see the social-psychological side of menstruation, a major paradigm shift needs to occur: It takes a great deal of thinking and discussion to cause a person to transfer focus from the medical model to the social-psychological model. Feminist therapists with more understanding of the social-psychological aspects of the menstrual cycle will be in the best position to help clients explore whether and how attitudes toward the experience of menstruation may be influencing development and interpersonal relating.

In this article, we have argued that our culture's negative messages about menstruation serve to reinforce a disconnection from menstruation for many girls and women and that women's varying attitudes toward and experiences with menstruation can serve as sources of disconnection among them. We suggest at least four major areas for therapeutic exploration of the impact of attitudes toward and experience of menstruation on women's development.

First, the mother-daughter relationship can be at risk, and especially at puberty, to the extent that mother and daughter do not talk about menstrual attitudes and experience, or have dissimilar experiences, and/or the mother dismisses the daughter's experience. No matter what age the client, a discussion of mother-daughter communication about menstruation could be explored. Questions to stimulate exploration might include, for example, Did your mother play a role in teaching you about menstruation? What messages about menstruation did your mother give to you? Did your mother share her own experience about menstruation? How did getting her period affect your relationship with your mother? Were you able to communicate your feelings about your period to your mother? Answers to these questions could provide insight into the degree to which a client may or may not have denied these parts of herself in order to stay in connection with her mother.

Second, relational problems or disconnections with other women that occur in friendships may essentially be a function of polar attitudes about menstrual topics that too often are based on an incomplete understanding of the variety of menstrual attitudes and experiences. Talking about the kinds of communication about menstruation the client has with her friends by using the following questions might be fruitful: Do you talk about your period with others such as your girlfriends? What kinds of things do you discuss? What has your experience been like with your period? If you had difficult times with your period, how have your friends reacted? How did they make you feel? Have you ever gotten the message that despite problems with your period, you should carry on as usual? If you have had no difficulties, what do you think about girls who have problems with their periods? A client's responses to these questions may reveal the extent to which menstruation is disconnecting her from other women.

Third, other areas of personal development and interpersonal relationship may be impacted, for example, self-doubt. As one young college-aged student put it recently, "Am I prone to be more moody because I am a woman? Are my strong feelings real or hormonal?" If a woman expresses anger premenstrually or during menstruation, she may get labeled a bitch, then feel guilty, and later apologize by blaming PMS or menstrual difficulties; or her concerns may be downplayed because she "takes back" any anger she expresses, or does not know how to express anger except in an extreme way. It may be important to assess the degree to which a client regards her menstrual experience as affecting her self-esteem, with the following questions: Thinking back to your adolescence, did getting your period change the way you thought of yourself? Did you see the experience as a loss or a gain? How did you feel then about being a female? Was the start of your period associated with sexuality or reproduction by your family or peers? If yes, how so? How did that make you feel? What kinds of things did you learn that you could (or could not) do while you had your period? Were there any traditional or religious beliefs surrounding a girl's period in your family? Do you think that PMS or your menstrual period affects your self-esteem? A discussion of these issues would reveal a client's attitudes toward menstruation and may reveal related negative self-constructs that have been created.

Fourth, menstrual attitudes and experience may also impact school or work. Taking time off and feeling guilty or grinning and bearing it may both lead to psychological stress. How does a client in this situation manage menstrual difficulties and workplace or school responsibilities? Does the client call in sick or miss school because of menstruation and then feel guilty for doing so? Or, does the client compensate and show up for work or school with possible negative consequences of performing poorly and/or feeling sick? An exploration of the strategies that a woman uses to cope with menstrual difficulties and manage her work or school load might lead to a reevaluation of her behavior and her negative self-constructs.

Although up to this point we have only discussed the influence of attitudes toward and experience with menstruation on relationships with women, other areas of impact may include intimate, friendship, and/or work-related interactions with men. We urge clinicians to broaden their view of the meaning of menstrual attitudes and experience in girls' and women's lives so that in turn, they may help clients diminish any negative self-constructs or disconnections in interpersonal relating associated with this most important aspect of being a female.

NOTES

1. Quotes in this section are from course assignments and/or course evaluations.

2. Despite recent news that HRT has not fulfilled its promise of a positive impact on the chronic health conditions that confront older women (Writing Group for the Women's Health Initiative Investigators, 2002), the debate about estrogen as an adjunct to women's health is far from over: Writing in the *New York Times Magazine*, Pachette (2002), suggested that the power of advertising creates a demand that overwhelms "science" and tells readers that while estrogen may be out of fashion now, give it another 10 or 20 years, and "women will still be there, lining up for the pill" (p. 11).

REFERENCES

Brooks-Gunn, J., & Ruble, D. N. (1977). The Menstrual Attitudes Questionnaire. *Psychosomatic Medicine, 42*, 503-512.

Brown, L., & Gilligan, C. (1992). *Meeting at the crossroads: Women's psychology and girls' development*. Cambridge, MA: Harvard University Press.

Caplan, P. J. (2001, May). Premenstrual mental illness: The truth about Sarafem. *The Network News, 26,* pp. 1, 5, 7.

Chrisler, J. C. (1988). Age, gender role orientation, and attitudes toward menstruation. *Psychological Reports, 63,* 827-834.

Chrisler, J. C. (1996). PMS as a culture-bound syndrome. In J. C. Chrisler, C. Golden, & P. D. Rozee (Eds.), *Lectures on the psychology of women* (pp. 106-121). Boston: McGraw Hill.

Chrisler, J. C., & Caplan, P. J. (2002). The strange case of Dr. Jekyll and Ms. Hyde: How PMS became a cultural phenomenon and psychiatric disorder. *Annual Review of Sex Research, 13,* 274-306.

Chrisler, J. C., & Johnston-Robledo, I. (2002). Raging hormones? Feminist perspectives on premenstrual syndrome and postpartum depression. In M. Ballou & L. S. Brown (Eds.), *Rethinking mental health and disorder: Feminist perspectives* (pp. 174-197). New York: Guilford.

Chrisler, J. C., & Levy, K. B. (1990). The media constructs a menstrual monster: A content analysis of PMS articles in the popular press. *Women & Health, 16*(2), 89-104.

Costos, D. (1995, June). *PMS as a vehicle for dividing women: An analysis of women's attitudes toward PMS and early education regarding menstruation.* Paper presented at the meeting of the Society for Menstrual Cycle Research, Montreal, Canada.

Costos, D., Ackerman, R., & Paradis, L. (2002). Recollections of menarche: Communication between mothers and daughters regarding menstruation. *Sex Roles, 46,* 83-101.

Coutinho, E. M., & Segal, S. J. (1999). *Is menstruation obsolete?* New York: Oxford University Press.

Crawford, M., & Unger R. (2000). *Women and gender: A feminist psychology* (3rd ed.). Boston: McGraw Hill.

Debold, E., Wilson, M., & Malave, I. (1993). *Mother daughter revolution: From betrayal to power.* New York: Addison-Wesley.

Delaney, J., Lupton, M. J., & Toth, E. (1988). *The curse: A cultural history of menstruation.* Champaign, IL: University of Illinois Press.

Egan, A. (1985). The selling of premenstrual syndrome. In S. Laws, V. Hey, & A. Eagan (Eds.), *Seeing red: The politics of premenstrual tension* (pp. 80-89). London: Hutchinson.

Erchull, M. I., Chrisler, J. C., Gorman, J. A., & Johnston-Robeldo, I. (2002). Education and advertising: A content analysis of commercially produced booklets about menstruation. *Journal of Early Adolescence, 22,* 455-474.

Gannon, L. (1998). The impact of medical and sexual politics on women's health. *Feminism & Psychology, 8,* 285-302.

Gillooly, J. (2004). Making menarche positive and powerful for both mother and daughter. *Women & Therapy, 27*(3/4), 23-35.

Golub, S. (1976). The effect of premenstrual anxiety and depression on cognitive function. *Journal of Personality and Social Psychology, 34,* 99-104.

Greene, A. L., & Adams-Price, C. (1990). Adolescents' secondary attachments to celebrity figures. *Sex Roles, 23*, 325-347.

Hey, V. (1985). Getting away with murder: PMT and the press. In S. Laws, V. Hey, & A. Eagan (Eds.), *Seeing red: The politics of premenstrual tension* (pp. 65-79). London: Hutchinson.

Houppert, K. (1999). *The curse: Confronting the last unmentionable taboo–menstruation.* New York: Farrar, Straus, & Giroux.

Kestenberg, J. (1967). Phases of adolescence, Part II: Prepuberty diffusion and reintegration. *Journal of the American Academy of Child Psychiatry, 6*, 577-611.

Koeske, R. (1980). Theoretical perspectives on menstrual cycle research: The relevance of attributional approaches for the perception and explanation of premenstrual emotionality. In A. J. Dan, E. A. Graham, & C. P. Beecher (Eds.), *The menstrual cycle: A synthesis of interdisciplinary research* (pp. 8-25). New York: Springer.

Koff, E. (1983). Through the looking glass of menarche: What the adolescent girl sees. In S. Golub (Ed.), *Menarche* (pp. 77-86). Lexington, MA: Lexington Books.

Koff, E., & Rierdan, J. (1995). Preparing girls for menstruation: Recommendations from adolescent girls. *Adolescence, 30*, 795-811.

Koff, E., Rierdan, J., & Silverstone, E. (1978). Changes in representation of body image as a function of menarcheal status. *Developmental Psychology, 14*, 635-642.

Koff, E., Rierdan, J., & Stubbs, M. L. (1990). Conceptions and misconceptions of the menstrual cycle. *Women & Health, 16*(3/4), 119-136.

Kruger, N., & Costos, D. (1997, June). *Gender role identity and attitude toward PMS.* Paper presented at the meeting of the Society for Menstrual Cycle Research, Chicago, IL.

Lee, J., & Sasser-Coen, J. (1996). *Blood stories: Menarche and the politics of the female body in contemporary U.S. society.* New York: Routledge.

MacPherson, K. (1981). Menopause as disease: The social construction of a metaphor. *Advances in Nursing Science, 3*, 95-113.

Martellock, A., & Costos, D. (1997, June). *Menopause as a culture bound syndrome.* Poster presented at the meeting of the Society for Menstrual Cycle Research, Chicago, IL.

Martin, E. (1987). *The woman in the body.* Boston: Beacon Press.

Miller, J. B., & Stiver, I. (1997). *The healing connection: How women form relationships in therapy and in life.* Boston: Beacon Press.

Nash, H. C., & Chrisler, J. C. (1997). Is a little (psychiatric) knowledge a dangerous thing? The impact of premenstrual dysphoric disorder on perceptions of premenstrual women. *Psychology of Women Quarterly, 21*, 315-322.

Pachette, A. (2002, July 28). Estrogen, after a fashion. *New York Times Magazine*, p. 11.

Parlee, M. B. (1974). Stereotypic beliefs about menstruation: A methodological note on the Moos Menstrual Distress Questionnaire and some new data. *Psychosomatic Medicine, 36*, 229-240.

Rierdan, J., & Koff, E. (1980). The psychological impact of menarche: Integrative versus disruptive changes. *Journal of Youth and Adolescence, 9*, 49-58.

Rierdan, J., Koff, E., & Flaherty, J. (1983). Guidelines for preparing girls for menstruation. *Journal of the American Academy of Child Psychiatry, 22,* 480-486.

Ruble, D. N. (1977). Premenstrual symptoms: A reinterpretation. *Science, 197,* 291-292.

Sommer, B. (1972). Menstrual cycle changes and intellectual performance. *Psychosomatic Medicine, 34,* 263-269.

Steinem, G. (1983). If men could menstruate. In G. Steinem (Ed.), *Outrageous acts and everyday rebellions* (pp. 366-369). New York: New American Library.

Stubbs, M. L. (1985). *Attitudes toward menstruation across the life span: The development of the Menstrual Experience and Attitude Questionnaire.* Unpublished doctoral dissertation, Brandeis University.

Stubbs, M. L. (1990). *Body talk: For parents of girls; for girls growing up; for parents of boys; for boys growing up.* Wellesley, MA: Centers for Research on Women.

Stubbs, M. L. (1993, June). *A rural perspective on the menstrual cycle.* Paper presented at the biennial meeting of the Society for Menstrual Cycle Research. Boston, MA.

Stubbs, M. L., Palmer, N., & Yandrich, A. (1999, June). *Teaching undergraduates about the menstrual cycle: Refining our pedagogy.* Paper presented at the biennial meeting of the Society for Menstrual Cycle Research. Tucson, AZ.

Stubbs, M. L., Rierdan, J., & Koff, E. (1989). Developmental differences in menstrual attitudes. *Journal of Early Adolescence, 9,* 480-489.

Whisnant, L., Brett, E., & Zegans, L. (1975). Implicit messages concerning menstruation in commercial educational materials prepared for young adolescent girls. *American Journal of Psychiatry, 132,* 815-820.

Williams, L. (1983). Beliefs and attitudes of young girls regarding menstruation. In S. Golub (Ed.), *Menarche: The transition from girl to woman* (pp. 139-148). Lexington, MA: Lexington Books.

Writing Group for the Women's Health Initiative Investigators. (2002). Risks and benefits of estrogen plus progestin in healthy postmenopausal women: Principal results from the Women's Health Initiative randomized controlled trial. *Journal of the American Medical Association, 288*(3), 321-333.

The Debate About PMDD and Sarafem: Suggestions for Therapists

Paula J. Caplan

SUMMARY. Complex and delicate issues of ethics and practice confront the feminist therapist in working with women who have been diagnosed, or have diagnosed themselves, as having "Premenstrual Dysphoric Disorder" (PMDD). The complexity arises from a combination of the fact that PMDD is an invented "mental illness" that has never been proven to exist, the aggressive marketing campaign created by pharmaceutical giant Eli Lilly for its drug Sarafem–which is actually Prozac–to treat this "disorder," and the reality that many women who are upset for good reasons believe that receiving the PMDD label is a sign that their reports of their feelings are believed. Suggestions are made for therapists to consider in grappling with this difficult confluence of facts and concerns. *[Article copies available for a fee from The Haworth Document Delivery Service: 1-800-HAWORTH. E-mail address: <docdelivery@haworthpress.com> Website: <http://www.HaworthPress.com> © 2004 by The Haworth Press, Inc. All rights reserved.]*

KEYWORDS. "Premenstrual Dysphoric Disorder," Sarafem, invented mental illness, therapists' dilemmas

Paula J. Caplan, PhD, is Research Professor (Adjunct) at Brown University, a clinical and research psychologist, and author of *They Say You're Crazy: How the World's Most Powerful Psychiatrists Decide Who's Normal.*

Address correspondence to: Paula J. Caplan, PhD, 26 Alpine St., Cambridge, MA 12138 (E-mail: Paula_Caplan@Brown.edu).

[Haworth co-indexing entry note]: "The Debate About PMDD and Sarafem: Suggestions for Therapists." Caplan, Paula J. Co-published simultaneously in *Women & Therapy* (The Haworth Press, Inc.) Vol. 27, No. 3/4, 2004, pp. 55-67; and: *From Menarche to Menopause: The Female Body in Feminist Therapy* (ed: Joan C. Chrisler) The Haworth Press, Inc., 2004, pp. 55-67. Single or multiple copies of this article are available for a fee from The Haworth Document Delivery Service [1-800-HAWORTH, 9:00 a.m. - 5:00 p.m. (EST). E-mail address: docdelivery@haworthpress.com].

The high-profit pharmaceutical companies are increasingly using the power of the mass media to persuade women that they have illnesses or disorders that require medication. But some of these "disorders" have not even been proven to exist. Few feminist therapists are medically trained or know much about drugs and their positive and negative effects on women's bodies. Furthermore, the power of people with medical degrees usually trumps that of non-MDs, whether in medical centers, mental health clinics, psychiatric residential facilities, the courts, or society in general. What, then, is a feminist therapist to do in the face of intense pressure to pathologize women and get them on medication? For some women in some situations, and with some conditions or problems, medication may be helpful, and drugs do not always have negative effects. But for the sake of women patients, feminist therapists must not let our lack of medical training silence us about the pathologizing of patients and the insistence of other professionals that women be medicated.

Women are telling their doctors–general practitioners, internal medicine specialists, obstetrician/gynecologists, psychiatrists–that they have diagnosed themselves with "Premenstrual Dysphoric Disorder" (PMDD), and they are asking for prescriptions for a drug they have seen advertised on television or in the pages of popular magazines. This is especially important because 84 percent of women who ask their physician for a drug by name leave the office with a prescription for it (O'Meara, 2001). The advertisements imply that women not only become bloated and experience chocolate cravings, breast tenderness, and irritability but actually become mentally ill and need to be treated with the "new," feminine-sounding drug called Sarafem. Sarafem is actually Prozac. Feminist and other women's Internet discussion lists have been buzzing with messages from women who feel insulted by ads that depict women as shrews. Neither the drugs nor the ads would exist without close interactions among the American Psychiatric Association, which creates the *Diagnostic and Statistical Manual of Mental Disorders (DSM)*,[1] Eli Lilly and other pharmaceutical companies, the media, and the women who sometimes feel physically bad and/or terribly upset–and long for their feelings to be taken seriously. But feminist therapists must not fall silent when the promoters of the concept of a premenstrual mental illness and of prescription drugs to treat that alleged illness tell our clients that labeling them mentally ill is the best or only way to show respect for their feelings.

THE HISTORY AND THE RESEARCH

In 1964, a British endocrinologist named Katharina Dalton coined the term "premenstrual syndrome" (PMS) and attached to it increasing numbers of "symptoms," both physical and psychological. Dalton was the prime mover in persuading both the medical community and laypeople that PMS was a real phenomenon, that husbands and children suffered terribly because their wives and mothers had "it," and that "it" went far beyond the cramps, bloating, and breast tenderness that had long been known to occur in some women in connection with the menstrual cycle (though one example of the confused thinking that plagues discussion of the topic is that cramps are often erroneously described as a PMS symptom, when in fact they occur during menstruation rather than before). Dalton's influence continues to be far-reaching, despite the incisive work done by, for instance, psychologist Mary Brown Parlee (1973) and biologist Anne Fausto-Sterling (1985) in revealing the multitude of methodological problems involved in trying to investigate almost anything about what people have called PMS. The concept of PMS was used to perpetuate the stereotype of women as overly emotional and unpredictable and thus needing to be reined in, if not by themselves then by drugs or some other means.

Thus, in the early 1980s, when influential *DSM* authors invented the alleged mental disorder now called PMDD, they did so in a cultural climate that already included a view of women as emotionally out of control (Chrisler, 2001), and the construct of "PMDD" rapidly became reified. Furthermore, there has been a long-standing tendency for doctors and others to dismiss women's medical complaints as imaginary; as a result, some women have been so relieved to have their physical discomfort and unpleasant feelings acknowledged that they have defended the label rather than asking whether they could, or deserve to, receive compassion and help without being diagnosed as mentally ill. Researcher Renay Tanner (quoted by O'Meara, 2001), among others (Chrisler & Caplan, 2002; Parlee, 1973; Fausto-Sterling, 1985), calls PMS/PMDD socially constructed diseases that are insulting to women. She has pointed out that the primary medication used to treat "PMDD" is also used by veterinarians to treat separation anxiety in dogs. And Tavris (1994) has pointed out that it is fairly easy to predict when premenstrual problems come in and out of public attention. She documented that "the idea that menstruation is a debilitating condition that makes women unfit for work . . . comes and goes in phase with women's participation in the labor market" (p. 139). The more that men need jobs, the stronger becomes the emphasis on women's unfitness for the workforce due to alleged menstrual cycle-related symptoms.

Research and clinical reports related to the premenstruum are extensive (see Caplan, McCurdy-Myers, and Gans, 1992, and Gold, Endicott, Parry, Severino, Stotland, and Frank, 1996, for reviews), but although most indicate that women have some physical problems at that time in the menstrual cycle, none provides proof that a premenstrual mental illness exists. O'Meara (2001) wrote that Eli Lilly's own literature revealed that there was no science to support the diagnosis. Indeed, if there were such an entity, and if its criteria were accurately identified and described in the *DSM*, the following study should have demonstrated it. Sheryle Gallant and her colleagues (Gallant, Popiel, Hoffman, Chakraborty, & Hamilton, 1992) took the symptoms listed for PMDD–then called Late Luteal Phase Dysphoric Disorder (LLPDD)–in the *DSM-III-R*–and asked three groups of people to document every day for two months which of the symptoms they experienced. They used this methodology because this was how the *DSM* authors said that PMDD should be diagnosed. The checklist was completed by women who reported severe premenstrual problems, women who reported no such problems, and men. Responses on the checklist failed to distinguish among the three groups; this study comes as close as one ever could to proving that PMDD does *not* exist.

The first inclusion of PMDD in the *DSM* was controversial and achieved in a disingenuous way. In reaction to an anti-PMDD protests at the 1986 conference of the Association for Women in Psychology and to protest by other groups that led to petitions and letters from individuals and organizations that represented more than six million people, some officials of the American Psychiatric Association proposed leaving PMDD out of the *DSM*. But psychiatrist Robert Spitzer, who headed the Task Force for the 1987 edition (*DSM-III-R*), proposed what he called a compromise: The category would go in a specially created appendix "for categories requiring further study."

It seemed like a victory for women that the label was given only provisional status, because the manual's main text is supposedly reserved for entities validated by scientific research. But once *DSM-III-R* was published, three things became clear. One, even though it was in the appendix, PMDD was given a five-digit code, a title, a list of symptoms, and a cutoff point (patients must have a specified number of symptoms to qualify for the label); i.e., it was presented exactly like the categories in the main text. Two, the appendix did not warn clinicians to avoid applying the label to patients. And three, the category was also listed in the main text (under Mood Disorders), despite the APA's claims that it was "only" in the appendix.

Seven years later, the authors of the 1994 edition (*DSM-IV*) continued to go to extraordinary lengths to push for inclusion of PMDD in the 4th edition. In the early 1990s, the LLPDD subcommittee undertook a massive literature review, after which they concluded that (1) very little research supported the existence of a premenstrual mental illness (that could be separated from the physical signs associated with PMS[2]); and (2) the most relevant research was preliminary and methodologically flawed. Nonetheless, the subcommittee reported to Allen Francis, who led the work on *DSM-IV*, that they could not reach a consensus about whether or not LLPDD should stay in the manual. Francis then chose two other people to make the final recommendation. He concealed their identities from the media and the public for months, and when their identities were revealed, neither turned out to be an expert in this field. Then *DSM* officials announced that the category (now called PMDD) would "continue" to be listed "only" in the provisional appendix.

When *DSM-IV* appeared, PMDD was not only in the appendix but also in the main text, now under "Depressive Disorders." Was it coincidence that A. John Rush, a specialist in depression, was one of the two people chosen to make the final recommendation? And one has to wonder why PMDD ended up in this category, because women need not be depressed in order to meet its criteria (one need only have a single mood symptom "marked" depression *or* anxiety, anger, or lability, plus four *physical* symptoms). This is a strange collection of symptoms for an alleged mental illness. Furthermore, any physician or psychotherapist who diagnoses a woman has to make a highly subjective judgment about whether her moods are "marked." That subjectivity might not be so worrisome were it not for the fact that the American Psychiatric Association uses as a major selling point what they describe as the impressive record of the manual in ensuring reliability and uniformity among therapists in their decisions about who meets the criteria for PMDD. In fact, diagnosticians' record of reliability in diagnosing PMDD is poor (see Caplan, 1995; Kirk & Kutchins, 1992).[3] Good reliability is an essential feature of validity, so it is interesting that in the *DSM-IV* LLPDD subcommittee report, Gold and her colleagues (1996) noted that "validity and clinical utility" were two of the basic issues that still needed to be addressed, but then they failed to address them. It is worrying that Gold et al. (1996) went on to write that "one measure of the utility of the LLPDD criteria is the considerable extent to which they have been accepted by both preclinical . . . and clinical . . . research groups" (p. 319). This is problematic because it has been well established that clinicians and researchers have often accepted and used diagnostic labels that were later considered to be ridiculous or even horrifying, such as the "psychiatric disorder" of drapetomania, which signified a slave's wish and attempts to get free (Caplan, 1995).

Related to the poor reliability and nonexistent validity of PMDD is that, as Gold et al. (1996) themselves reported, many studies of PMDD include the instruction to women to rate their symptoms daily for one menstrual cycle, even though in the *DSM* itself it is specified that daily ratings are to be kept for at least *two* cycles. Furthermore, Gold et al. (1996) noted that "Multiple hormone samples are needed throughout the cycle to establish . . . menstrual cycle phase. [But] very few studies have done this" (p. 321). This is particularly problematic because, although some women's cycles are regular, others' cycles vary considerably. If, then, a researcher finds that a woman's ratings show that she feels more upset on some days than on others, it is impossible to verify whether she was actually "premenstrual" (i.e., in the luteal phase) in terms of her hormone levels. Thus, further confusion and uncertainty are added to the search for truth about the category because of researchers' unstandardized use of the criteria and their failure to investigate at what point in her cycle a given woman's mood changes may occur. In fact, according to Gold et al. (1996), in a study in which morning blood samples were drawn, no diagnosis-related changes were found in any of the hormones. Despite the widespread acceptance of the notion that raging hormones render teenage girls and premenstrual, perimenopausal, and even postmenopausal women utterly irrational and hysterical, there is simply no evidence that directly connects hormone levels to mood or behavior. That does not mean that the way one *interprets or deals with* hormonal changes cannot have an impact on mood or behavior, but there is no proof of a direct connection.

A further reflection of the closed-society functioning of *DSM* groups is that some consultants to the LLPDD subcommittee (including me) were never notified of meeting dates nor given some of the crucial information and data the subcommittee possessed. Often, our feedback was solicited after relevant deadlines had passed. (After the publication of *DSM-III-R*, I contacted Francis and offered to send him the reviews that my students and I planned to write. He invited me to join the subcommittee, assuring me that "this time" decisions about the manual would be based on scientific evidence.)

From the beginning, the only recommended psychiatric therapy for PMDD has been antidepressants, usually fluoxetine (Prozac). Although dietary and exercise changes or participation in self-help groups are sometimes recommended, the big push has been for drugs. This push was made despite Lilly's apparently having provided no evidence that any beneficial effects on women diagnosed with PMDD are due to anything other than a masking of discomfort by the drug (O'Meara, 2001).

Despite being sent documentation that this diagnostic label has harmed women, from child-custody challenges (Dalton, 1979, and Mullen, 1980, both cited by Gold et al., 1996) to suicide attempts, LLPDD subcommittee chair Judith Gold has publicly denied knowing of any reports of harm. In fact, Gold et al. (1996) wrote that an important question related to LLPDD was "What are the potential social, forensic, and occupational risks of including the LLPDD diagnosis in *DSM-IV*? How would the existence of these risks be assessed?" (p. 319). These are certainly important questions, and it is troubling that the *DSM* people failed to address them. One important attempt to answer these questions was a study by Nash and Chrisler (1997), who found that the very existence of the concept of PMDD has resulted in women's perceptions of what happens to them before their periods becoming more pathological than before PMDD was invented.

Furthermore, O'Meara (2001) reported that a draft of proposed "Precaution and Adverse Reactions" sections for the Prozac package insert included the sentence "Mania and psychosis may be precipitated in susceptible patients by antidepressant therapy," but that sentence was never included in the actual inserts. Also according to O'Meara (2001), an Eli Lilly employee in Germany expressed concern in a memo about Lilly's description as an "overdose" what a physician reported as a suicide attempt and as "depression" what a physician reported as suicidal ideation. In fact, according to O'Meara (2001), although Lilly has consistently denied that Prozac can cause suicidal thoughts, the company obtained a patent to develop what apparently would be a pharmaceutical variation that would eliminate Prozac's potential to cause suicidal thoughts.

In June 1999, with the patent on Prozac about to expire, its manufacturer, Eli Lilly & Co., organized a roundtable discussion that was attended by many of the PMDD subcommittee members. If Prozac were approved for a different "mental illness," it would extend the patent for some time, which would be an economic boon to the company. This is because the Food and Drug Administration does not grant approval for a particular drug to be prescribed for any disease or disorder but only for a particular one. Prozac was initially approved by the FDA for treatment of depression. If Lilly could show that Prozac was beneficial for treating some other condition, they might get additional FDA approval and an extension of their patent on Prozac. Lilly appears to have presented PMDD to the FDA as though it were a real entity. An article presented as the state-of-the-science result of the Lilly-sponsored roundtable titled "Is Premenstrual Dysphoric Disorder a Distinct Clinical Entity?" (Endicott et al., 1999) was published in the *Journal of Women's Health and Gender-Based Medicine*. Presumably recalling their own description of pre-*DSM-IV* research as sparse and methodologically poor (e.g., see Gold et al., 1996), the authors claimed that more recent evidence proved PMDD to be "real" and Prozac to be an effective treatment. But only a tiny number of the articles cited were truly post-*DSM-IV* research, and those provided no evidence that a premenstrual mental illness exists. Much of the roundtable article (Endicott et al., 1999) constituted a promotion of Prozac through statements that Prozac improves symptoms of women with "PMDD." Certainly, if Prozac is given to any group of depressed or upset people, some will feel better. But that reveals nothing about the causes of their upset and, in this case, it doesn't prove that the upset is related to menstrual cycle-related changes. Furthermore, as Tavris has said, if women are depressed, they should be treated for depression (Tavris, 1992), not for "PMDD." The report of Gold et al. (1996) that there is significant overlap and "comorbidity" with other mental disorders supports the idea that what is being called PMDD is quite likely one or more other real or alleged mental disorders. In fact, Gold et al. wrote that most studies of co-morbidity "have failed to clearly differentiate women with LLPDD alone from those with exacerbations of ongoing mental disorders or concurrent comorbid mental disorders" (p. 327) and that few articles were found in which that distinction was made.

The FDA's Psychopharmacological Drugs Advisory Committee (PDAC) met on November 3, 1999. There, representatives of Eli Lilly & Co. brought PMDD subcommittee member Jean Endicott, first author of the roundtable paper, to speak. According to the minutes, there was consensus among committee members that PMDD is a recognized and well-defined clinical entity and that there are accepted diagnostic criteria for it. The PDAC voted "yes" unanimously on the question "Has the sponsor provided evidence from more than one adequate and well controlled clinical investigation that supports the conclusion that fluoxetine [the active ingredient in both Prozac and Sarafem] is effective for the treatment of Premenstrual Dysphoric Disorder?" and "no" on the question of whether Prozac caused harm to people with PMDD. It's hard to imagine what the outcome of that vote might have been without the assistance of Dr. Endicott and the roundtable article.

Why was the FDA's decision bad for women? First, Sarafem is Prozac renamed and repackaged in the "feminine" colors of purple and pink.[4] Many women for whom Sarafem is prescribed won't know that, and might choose not to take a mind-altering drug if they did know. Second, Prozac has negative effects on many people. By promoting fluoxetine for premenstrual problems, Lilly stands to broaden its use to millions of women, many of whom will not benefit from the drug. Negative effects such as nausea, insomnia, headache, dizziness, nervousness, increased appetite, and sexual dysfunction (Gold et al., 1996) might be acceptable to women with severe depression–not to mention the (probably less common) overdosing and suicidal ideation described above–but they might be unacceptable for women diagnosed with PMDD who have milder, more manageable, or primarily physical symptoms. Safe, effective options exist for women with troublesome premenstrual or menstrual problems, including calcium supplementation (which in the roundtable article was only briefly mentioned and certainly not pushed as treatment for PMDD as Prozac was, despite the similar levels of effectiveness reported for calcium and for Prozac), cognitive therapy (including questioning the assumption that one's anger is never justified), and self-help groups, as well as exercise, and dietary changes (Caplan, 1995). Pirie and Smith (1992) have found that merely talking about their "PMS" with other women reduces the severity of symptoms by 40-50 percent. This is impressively close to the 50-65 percent improvement rate claimed for treatment with Prozac and related drugs (Endicott et al., 1999). The FDA's decision to accept Lilly's description of Prozac as effective for "PMDD" exacerbates the misleading and dangerous assumption that this condition even exists. The first Sarafem commercial, which showed a woman frantic because she couldn't extract a shopping cart from a row of carts, included a voiceover that warned women that they might think they have PMS when they really have PMDD. Subsequent ads have continued to convey that message, which conflates PMS with PMDD and uses the alleged pervasiveness of PMS as a foothold to imply that PMDD is also very common.

The FDA is not the only federal government agency that has taken part in the focusing on Sarafem. Carmody, Collins, Dyer, and Frosino (2002) reported that when a woman telephoned the National Institutes of Mental Health and asked for information about resources in the Boston area about PMS, she was referred to the Sarafem Website.

The problem with PMDD is not the women who report that they have premenstrual emotional problems; the problem is with diagnosis of PMDD itself. Feminist researchers have found that women diagnosed (by professionals or by themselves) as having PMDD are significantly more likely than other women to be or have been in upsetting life situations, such as being battered or being mistreated at work (see Caplan, 1995) or to have experienced sexual abuse or other trauma (Golding & Taylor, 1996; Golding, Taylor, Menard, & King, 2000; Taylor, 1999). Ian Tummon (1993), an obstetrician-gynecologist who has suggested (Tummon & Kramer, 1994) that even the term "PMS" no longer be used, reported that when his women patients begin an office visit by saying, "Doctor, I have terrible PMS," they never again mention PMS during the rest of the session. Instead, he wrote, they spend the whole time talking about the way their husbands abuse them or about their 14-year-old children who won't come home at night. To label these women mentally disordered–and send the message that their problems are individual, psychological ones–hides the real, external sources of their trouble. Furthermore, for women who need and want psychotherapy, medication can mask important feelings and thus inhibit the work of therapy. And it is troubling that the PMDD label implies that it is hormonally caused, although a memo to the LLPDD subcommittee from its chair, Judith Gold, noted that the symptoms listed under PMDD might not be due to hormonal factors (Gold, 1993).

The creation of Sarafem has extended Lilly's patent on Prozac, thus adding untold profits to its bottom line. This is an example of a company's taking cynical advantage of the legal and regulatory system to increase its profits at the expense of women's health.

SUGGESTIONS FOR THERAPISTS

It is common now for women to diagnose themselves as having "PMS" or "PMDD," a practice promoted by the multitude of books written for laypeople about "PMS" that have done much to perpetuate the stereotype of premenstrual women as utterly out of control (Chrisler, 2001). Furthermore, an unknown but probably large percentage of the women who believe they have "PMS" or "PMDD" are now taking Sarafem, quite possibly unaware of the profoundly disturbing research information and/or of the understanding that a feminist perspective brings to the subject. Chrisler (2001) has noted that it is important for health care practitioners to know what their clients are likely to know or believe about syndromes described as menstrually related. Psychotherapists need to learn how much their clients know, find a way to make clear their respect for their clients, and also convey information their clients might or might not want to hear. All of the following suggestions should be considered in the following context: Some of these clients will have only emotional-social problems, some will have physical ones, and some will have both.

As with any patient who requests psychotherapy for emotional or physical complaints, it is important for both ethical and legal reasons to make sure that they have thorough medical workups–by internists and perhaps by neurologists. In this way, one can reduce the chances that one is engaged in a "talking cure" with a patient whose mood changes and/or physical problems are caused by a brain tumor, temporal lobe seizures, or the effects of even a long-ago traumatic automobile or athletic accident. However, medical doctors often miss physiologically based problems. For instance, few are aware that even a mild or moderate car accident can seriously intensify the muscle pain and tightness of fibromyalgia. For this reason, a responsible therapist will make it a point to seek out and refer clients to the most knowledgeable, local physicians and alternative practitioners (in my experience, chiropractors are more likely than physicians to be aware of the connection between an accident and the intensification of fibromyalgia). If the matter of "PMDD" comes up after you have already begun the psychotherapy, you can urge that these workups be done at that time.

In any case, because people who seek psychotherapy are usually undergoing intense anguish, sadness, fear, shame, or some combination of these, it is essential to listen carefully to the woman's descriptions of what she presents as her

"PMDD"-related problems. Be sure to indicate that you believe that she is experiencing these problems.

Before going any farther, the therapist will want to address the following matter: How does a therapist who shares my opinion of "PMDD" deal with the concern that she is trying to manipulate the patient into sharing that view? In my opinion, to *inform* the patient that the material reported above exists and to *offer* to tell her how to find it differs little or not at all from the longstanding practice of giving patients books about feminist research and analysis or stories about key matters in their lives. Furthermore, for years, feminist therapists have considered it important to help the patient understand how the problems that brought her to therapy may have been aggravated or even created by the messages, social arrangements, and power distribution of a woman-hating society (Robbins & Siegel, 1983). Related to "PMDD," for instance, is the fact that there are no data to suggest that women are angrier or more aggressive than men on a cyclical basis (Caplan, 1995), and yet "PMDD" is used to pathologize women's anger.

Each therapist must decide for herself whether she believes it is appropriate and therapeutic to offer clients information and her own viewpoint. Another consideration is that *failing to disclose* relevant knowledge or her own view might be considered unethical and may cause even a well-intentioned therapist to manipulate the client in ways that move her toward sharing the therapist's view *without the client, and maybe the therapist, being able to monitor that process consciously.*

A related concern is how to convey one's respect for the patient when informing her of the evidence that there is no such thing as the "mental illness" she believes she has and that the drug she is taking may be inappropriate or even harmful. It is helpful to begin the conversation by addressing the importance of giving people the opportunity to *choose* how to conduct their lives. Then one can point out to clients that one choice is whether or not to hear about material that conflicts with their current beliefs, attitudes, or practices. The therapist can make it clear that she is raising this subject because she feels strongly that people should be able to make choices that are based on complete information and because she respects the clients' ability to consider and evaluate information.

If a client expresses a wish to be more fully informed, the therapist can offer to suggest reading material and/or to describe her own understanding of the information and why it matters. If a client wants to do some reading, one option is to give her this article (because I have tried to keep it clear and jargon-free), and mention that it includes references so that she can go to the research reports and evaluate them herself if she likes. Or one could give her a list of relevant references. Then it's helpful to offer to talk with her about the thoughts, feelings, and questions that result from her reading of this material or hearing of your description of it. And in this connection it is also helpful to communicate Parlee's (1994) observation that to conclude that suffering is not biologically based should not be to conclude that it is not real.

If she rejects your offer of information or, after receiving that information, continues to maintain that she has "PMDD" and continues to take Sarafem, what do you do? If you believe that this will seriously impede her progress in therapy–for instance, if she sticks with the belief that all of the "unfeminine" feelings she has, such as anger, result from her "PMDD"–you are obligated to tell her that, just as you would with any other major impediment to therapy. Otherwise, you will continue to receive payment for a service that you doubt you can provide. Similarly, if you learn from a patient that she is doing something that could hurt her, it is your ethical obligation to tell her of that concern. That can be done as a statement of your worry, or it can be done by pointing out her options (to believe or not believe she has "PMDD," to take or not take Sarafem) and exploring with her the very different courses those different options would lead her to follow. For instance, if attributing her anger to a mental disorder keeps her from telling her husband what else might be making her angry, then what advantages and/or disadvantages accrue to her from doing this? What impact might her different options have on her children or other loved ones? Related to this is one of the most common of feminist therapists' practices, which is to raise clients' awareness of the powerful effects created by the belief that a good woman is never angry. One form of that practice is to try to explore with a client the possibility that PMDD might be important to her because it allows her to say, "I can't help being angry. Blame my hormones, not me" (Caplan, 1995).

If a client continues with a course of treatment that worries you but does not seem likely to interfere seriously with your work with her, it will be important to ensure that she arranges for you and the other treating professional to receive regular updates about how each other's treatment is going. It is also crucial for you to make sure that you are informed about what kinds of negative effects can result from other treatments your client is receiving, so that you can be on alert for them. And, as always, it is part of a responsible feminist therapist's work to inform clients that the fact that government agencies may be approving and/or recommending particular treatments is no guarantee that they are safe and that the plethora of popular books whose authors claim to be telling the truth about premenstrual problems and treatments is no guarantee that they are right (Chrisler, 2001). It is also important to tell clients about what has been helpful to other people, including not only drugs but also self-help groups, cognitive behavior therapy, and changes in diet and nutrition.

Threading one's way through this morass of considerations and principles seems complex and delicate precisely because it is unavoidably so (see Pope & Vasquez, 1998, for discussion of ethical principles). But the subject increasingly arises for women and therefore for feminist therapists. My final suggestion, then, is to take every opportunity to raise these concerns and dilemmas with other therapists and with nontherapists (obviously protecting patients' confidentiality) and see what they have to say, showing that you are grappling with them and have no easy answers. Therapists will probably be relieved to find that they are not the only ones who find this a difficult ground to tread, and together you may make considerable headway.

NOTES

1. At the request of Allen Francis, head of the *DSM-IV* Task Force, I served as a consultant to the PMDD group for *DSM-IV*, and saw how the *DSM* was being put together. I was profoundly troubled by what I learned about the process, including the way decisions about what was and was not normal were often made on political grounds rather than scientific ones and the ways that scientific research was often distorted or ignored. I (1995) wrote *They Say You're Crazy: How the World's Most Powerful Psychiatrists Decide Who's Normal* to make that story, with documentation, available to both therapists and patients, most of whom had no idea that the *DSM* was not the scientifically based compendium it was alleged to be by its publisher, the American Psychiatric Association.

2. Almost no one bothers any more to distinguish PMS from PMDD, although the *DSM* authors had always claimed that PMDD was a label for only a tiny proportion of women with extremely severe *emotional* symptoms. In all the decades before the category of PMDD was thought up, "PMS" was generally used to refer to physical symptoms such as bloating, breast tenderness, food cravings, and mood changes that women might find troubling or embarrassing but that were not commonly described as constituting a mental illness. Now "PMDD" is often used to subsume what was called "PMS." This is especially blatant in the advertisements for Sarafem (Chrisler & Caplan, 2002).

3. Gold et al. (1996) reported that "women are expected to exhibit affect and change affect more easily than men. The distinction between affective responsiveness and 'emotional lability,' a *DSM-III-R* criterion for the LLPDD disorder, cannot be made with validity or reliability (Verbrugge, 1979)" (p. 375).

4. O'Meara (2001) reported that an Eli Lilly marketing associate refused to acknowledge that Sarafem is just Prozac repackaged or that its color was changed to market it for a "mental disorder" that had never before existed.

REFERENCES

American Psychiatric Association. (1987). *Diagnostic and statistical manual of mental disorders-III-R*. Washington, D.C.: American Psychiatric Association.

American Psychiatric Association. (1994). *Diagnostic and statistical manual of mental disorders-IV*. Washington, D.C.: American Psychiatric Association.

Caplan P. J. (1995). *They say you're crazy: How the world's most powerful psychiatrists decide who's normal*. Reading, MA: Addison Wesley.

Caplan, P. J., McCurdy-Myers, J., & Gans, M. (1992). Should "premenstrual syndrome" be called a psychiatric abnormality? *Feminism and Psychology, 2*, 27-44.

Carmody, C., Collins, B., Dyer, M., & Frosino, T. (2002). Who is being served? The pros, cons, and social implications for the inclusion of PMDD in the *DSM*. Boston: University of Massachusetts, Counseling Department.

Chrisler, J. C. (2001). *How to regain your control and balance: The "pop" approach to PMS*. Unpublished manuscript.

Chrisler, J. C., & Caplan, P. J. (2002). The strange case of Dr. Jekyll and Ms. Hyde: How PMS became a cultural phenomenon and a psychiatric disorder. *Annual Review of Sex Research, 13*, 274-306.

Dalton, K. (1964). *The premenstrual syndrome.* Springfield, IL: Charles C. Thomas.

Endicott, J., Amsterdam, J., Eriksson, E., Frank, E., Freeman, E., Hirschfield, R., Ling, F., Parry, B., Pearlstein, T., Rosenbaum, J., Rubinow, D., Schmidt, P., Severino, S., Steiner, M., Stewart, D., & Thys-Jacobs, S. (1999). Is Premenstrual Dysphoric Disorder a distinct clinical entity? *Journal of Women's Health and Gender-Based Medicine, 8,* 663-679.

Fausto-Sterling, A. (1985). *Myths of gender: Biological theories about women and men.* New York: Basic Books.

Gallant, S., Popiel, D., Hoffman, D., Chakraborty, P., & Hamilton, J. (1992). Using daily ratings to confirm Premenstrual Syndrome/Late Luteal Phase Dysphoric Disorder. Part II. What makes a 'real' difference? *Psychosomatic Medicine, 54,* 167-81.

Gold, J. (1993, March 8). Memo to LLPDD subcommittee.

Gold, J., Endicott, J., Parry, B., Severino, S., Stotland, N., & Frank, E. (1996). Late Luteal Phase Dysphoric Disorder. In T. Widiger, A. Frances, H. A. Pincus, R. Ross, M. B. First, & W. W. Davis (Eds.), *DSM-IV Sourcebook* (Vol. 2, pp. 317-94). Washington, D.C.: American Psychiatric Association.

Golding, J. M., & Taylor, D. (1996). Sexual assault history and premenstrual distress in two general population samples. *Journal of Women's Health, 5,* 143-52.

Golding, J. M., Taylor, D. L., Menard, L., & King, M. J. (2000). Prevalence of sexual abuse history in a sample of women seeking treatment for premenstrual syndrome. *Journal of Psychosomatic Obstetrics and Gynecology, 21,* 69-80.

Kirk, S., & Kutchins, H. (1992). *The selling of DSM: The rhetoric of science in psychiatry.* New York: Aldine DeGruyter.

Nash, H. C., & Chrisler, J. C. (1997). Is a little (psychiatric) knowledge a dangerous thing? The impact of premenstrual dysphoric disorder on perceptions of premenstrual women. *Psychology of Women Quarterly, 21,* 315-322.

O'Meara, K. P. (2001, April 30). Misleading medicine. *Insight on the News,* p. 10.

Parlee, M. B. (1994, June 17). Personal communication.

Parlee, M. B. (1973). The Premenstrual Syndrome. *Psychological Bulletin, 80,* 454-65.

Pirie, M., & Smith, L. H. (1992, December). Coping with PMS: A women's health center has success with a life skills model. *Canadian Nurse,* pp. 24-25, 46.

Pope, K. S., & Vasquez, M. J. T. (Eds.). (1998). *Ethics in psychotherapy and counselling: A practical guide.* San Francisco: Jossey Bass.

Robbins, J. H., & Siegel, R. J (Eds.). (1983). *Women changing therapy: New assessments, values, and strategies in feminist therapy.* New York: The Haworth Press, Inc.

Tavris, C. (1992). *The mismeasure of woman.* New York: Simon and Schuster.

Taylor, D. (1999). Effectiveness of professional-peer group treatment: Symptom management for women with PMS. *Research in Nursing & Health, 22,* 496-511.

Tummon, I. (1993, June). Personal communication.

Tummon, I., & Kramer, B. (1994). Time to discard the diagnosis of premenstrual syndrome? *Journal of the Society of Obstetricians and Gynecologists, 16,* 1565-70.

Verbrugge, L. M. (1979). Female illness rates and illness behavior. *Women & Health, 4,* 61-79.

Abortion and Mental Health:
What Therapists Need to Know

Lisa Rubin
Nancy Felipe Russo

SUMMARY. Unwanted pregnancy and abortion are common life events, and therapists are likely to work with clients who experience them. Legal abortion currently entails little physical or mental health risk; most women currently cope effectively with these life events without need of clinical intervention. But current abortion politics include efforts to make abortion a more threatening, stressful, and stigmatized experience and to create a "postabortion syndrome." Using a stress and coping framework, we examine how antiabortion activists spread myths and misinformation aimed at women's appraisal processes, and discuss approaches therapists can use to enhance women's strategies for coping with abortion. We also discuss specific issues and useful techniques for counseling about abortion concerns, including cultural sensitivity and strategies for promoting positive sexual health. *[Article copies available for a fee from The Haworth Document Delivery Service: 1-800-HAWORTH. E-mail address: <docdelivery@haworthpress.com>*

Lisa Rubin, MA, is a doctoral student in clinical psychology at Arizona State University. Nancy Felipe Russo, PhD, is Regent's Professor of Psychology and Women's Studies at Arizona State University.

Address correspondence to: Nancy Felipe Russo, Psychology, Box 871104, Arizona State University, Tempe, AZ 85287-1104 (E-mail: nancy.russo@asu.edu or lisa.rubin@asu.edu).

[Haworth co-indexing entry note]: "Abortion and Mental Health: What Therapists Need to Know." Rubin, Lisa, and Nancy Felipe Russo. Co-published simultaneously in *Women & Therapy* (The Haworth Press, Inc.) Vol. 27, No. 3/4, 2004, pp. 69-90; and: *From Menarche to Menopause: The Female Body in Feminist Therapy* (ed: Joan C. Chrisler) The Haworth Press, Inc., 2004, pp. 69-90. Single or multiple copies of this article are available for a fee from The Haworth Document Delivery Service [1-800-HAWORTH, 9:00 a.m. - 5:00 p.m. (EST). E-mail address: docdelivery@haworthpress.com].

10.1300/J015v27n03_06

KEYWORDS. Abortion, postabortion syndrome, unwanted pregnancy, pregnancy termination, abortion counseling

The sociocultural environment in which women make abortion decisions reinforces ambivalence at best, and at worst introduces negative thoughts and feelings with which women might not otherwise be troubled.

–Jeanne Parr Lemkau (1988, p. 461)

INTRODUCTION

Unintended pregnancy and abortion are common events in women's lives. According to the Alan Guttmacher Institute (2002), nearly half of pregnancies in the United States are unintended. In addition to the fact that unwanted pregnancy is a stressful experience in and of itself, the highest rates of such pregnancies occur for women at risk for stress and mental health problems associated with poverty and discrimination (i.e., young, poor, unmarried, Black, or Hispanic women), and who have less access to resources for dealing with such problems. A little over half of unintended pregnancies are terminated by abortion. With approximately 1.3 million abortions annually, abortion continues to play an essential role in enabling women in the United States to time, space, and limit their births (Alan Guttmacher Institute, 2002). Given these "facts of life," therapists are very likely to work with clients who have had or face unwanted pregnancies, and some of those women will have experienced abortion.

Distress in a woman who has experienced an unwanted pregnancy, regardless of how the pregnancy is resolved, is not surprising. Further, sometimes women initially want to become pregnant but ultimately seek abortion because of changed circumstances (e.g., divorce, illness, discovery of a fetal defect). In such cases the decision-making process appears to be more stressful (David, 1985).

Abortion is extremely safe compared to its alternatives: the risk of death associated with childbirth is about 10 times as high as that associated with abortion. Risk of death associated with abortion increases with the length of pregnancy: at 8 or fewer weeks about 1 woman dies for every 530,000 abortions; at 16-20 weeks the figure is 1 woman per 17,000 abortions. For the 1% of women who have abortions at 21 or more weeks the figure is 1 woman per

6,000 abortions. Late abortions involve a more risky, painful, and traumatic process, and do not represent the experience of the approximately 90% of women who obtain abortions during the first trimester (12 or fewer weeks of gestation; Alan Guttmacher Institute, 2002). In general, the discussion here focuses on abortion during the first trimester of pregnancy.

When abortion is legal, its risk for severe psychological problems appears comparable to that of giving birth (Wilmoth, de Alteriis, & Bussell, 1992). Nonetheless, a minority of women experience severe negative postabortion responses (Adler, David, Major, Roth, Russo, & Wyatt, 1990, 1992; Russo, 1992; Denious & Russo, 2000). Therapists must be prepared to provide appropriate support and mental health services for women when such reactions occur (Kahn-Edrington, 1979; Lemkau, 1988; Denious & Russo, 2000).

Although information in this article may be useful for counselors in family planning centers and abortion clinics, our intended audience is psychotherapists who have not received specialized training in abortion issues. All therapists are trained to help clients cope with stressful life events, but the political context of abortion and the current activities of antiabortion activists complicate the therapeutic process. When dealing with value-laden, politicized issues such as abortion, knowledge of how the larger social context affects clients' mental health and well-being is indispensable for achieving therapeutic goals. In this article we discuss therapeutic issues that are shaped by the current political context and provide information useful for counseling women who have had or are thinking about having an abortion.

Viewpoints and Values

Whether or not to terminate an unwanted pregnancy is a deeply personal decision made even more difficult by the fact that abortion is a value-laden, controversial topic. A first step toward providing women with effective therapy is for therapists to be clear on their own viewpoints and values. In this article, we conceptualize unwanted pregnancy and abortion from a stress and coping perspective. We assume that the interaction of situational (e.g., social, political, economic, and cultural considerations) and intrapsychic factors (e.g., personal traits and resilience, cognitive appraisals, and coping strategies) is what ultimately determines mental health outcomes (Lazarus & Folkman, 1984; Russo & Green, 1993).

From this perspective, a woman's appraisal of her life events–their meaning to her–plays a key role in determining her mental health. Further, her coping resources–psychological and social–are critical determinants as well. Consequently, women's responses to unwanted pregnancy terminated by a voluntarily chosen legal abortion can range from feelings of empowerment and satisfaction from successfully dealing with a major life challenge to guilt and shame for not having psychological, social, and/or economic resources to commit to a child.

A major goal of therapy in this context is to reveal specific links that lead to positive and negative mental health outcomes for each particular client as a prelude to moving the client on to a healthier psychological state. Doing this requires that the therapist recognize and set aside preconceived notions about the meaning of abortion and women's responses to it. Therapists must be clear about their values with themselves and with their clients. If a therapist cannot do this, the responsible thing is to refer clients to someone who can.

As 43% of women are expected to have at least one abortion by the time they are 45 years old (Alan Guttmacher Institute, 2002), it is likely that many therapists will have had abortions themselves. We need to recognize that responses to reproductive events such as unwanted pregnancy and abortion range widely; we cannot assume that because therapist and client both have had an abortion that they have had the same experience.

Therapists with feminist values recognize that women's lives often involve stressful choices and seek to provide clients with the information, skills, support, and confidence to be active and effective decision makers more in control of their fate. They understand that having an unwanted pregnancy and abortion is typically a stressful event but that most women cope effectively with the situation. Nonetheless, for some women, the effects of unwanted pregnancy and abortion are more profound and serious. If they do not receive help from unbiased therapists they will be ripe for manipulation by antiabortion organizations seeking to exploit their vulnerabilities to advance an antiabortion political agenda. In such cases, the therapist's role involves exploring the meaning and context of women's feelings and providing women with the information, insights, and support they need to move on with their lives. In this context, effective therapy requires equipping clients with knowledge and skills to make their own responsible life choices free from manipulation and coercion.

To achieve therapeutic goals, clients need to understand where their ideas about the meaning of abortion have come from and to reevaluate the bases for those ideas (for examples of some of the issues that women bring to therapy, see peaceafterabortion.com). To help clients, therapists must understand the politics of abortion and the misinformation and myth-making involved in antiabortion attempts to make abortion a stigmatized and stressful experience.

THE POLITICAL CONTEXT

When society shames us for our abortions, it affects how we mourn, discuss, and accept them.

–Eve Kushner (1997, p. 9)

Strategies antiabortion activists use to make abortion a stigmatized and stressful experience have included intimidation of patients, harassment of staff, vandalism, bombings, and murder of physicians. Picketing of abortion clinics is a threatening act in this context of terrorism. Women are photographed and followed, screamed at, called names such as "baby-killer," and told that abortion will give them cancer, cause infertility, and make them spiritually and mentally ill. They are shown grotesque pictures of body parts of fetuses of unknown origin that are gestationally well advanced beyond the time the vast majority of women have legal abortions. They are told that the fetus experienced pain and that they have denied access of their aborted child to heaven. In addition to threatening and stigmatizing women, such activities undermine feelings of self-efficacy for coping with an abortion, deter social support, foster shame and guilt, and create barriers that inhibit access to this important means for coping with the stress of unwanted pregnancy. The resulting decrements in mental health can then be used as further evidence of abortion's injurious effects. In addition to undermining women's mental health and well-being directly, such tactics result in unwanted childbearing, with all of the negative long-term physical and mental health consequences that such childbearing entails for women, their families, and society (David, Dytrych, Matejcek, & Schüller, 1988; Russo, 1992).

In 1973 when the U.S. Supreme Court legalized abortion in *Roe v. Wade*, it set the stage for the pregnant woman's psychological status to assume a larger role in what has been called the "abortion wars" (Solinger, 1998). Beyond contributing to efforts to overturn *Roe v. Wade*, construction of a postabortion syndrome plays a central role in a complex strategy designed to make abortion inaccessible by holding physicians "fully liable for all the physical, psychological, and spiritual injuries they inflict on women" (Elliot Institute, 1997). This strategy goes beyond harassing doctors with frivolous legal proceedings and raising the cost of malpractice insurance. Activists attempt to pass legislation making physicians civilly and criminally liable for damages from such "injuries," damages that are ineligible for malpractice insurance coverage.

Antiabortion advocates allege that "postabortion syndrome" is a type of post-traumatic stress disorder (PTSD), though no scientific basis exists for applying a PTSD framework to understand women's emotional responses to a voluntarily obtained legal abortion. Abortion is a common life event, and women do not typically exhibit severe negative responses during or after having one, particularly if the abortion is legal and the pregnancy early. Women do not typically fear for their lives during a legal abortion (and reasonably so, given it is safer than a penicillin shot), a basic criterion for assigning a PTSD diagnosis. When women do experience extreme distress, the pattern of their responses during and after legal abortion does not fit a PTSD profile. That is, the point of highest distress is *before* the abortion rather than during and just after it, as is characteristic of responses to violent experiences in war or being raped. Distress levels begin to drop after the abortion and continue to diminish over several months. Studies of other life stressors suggest that women who show no evidence of severe negative responses after a stressful event are unlikely to develop significant psychological problems in the future in conjunction with that event (Adler et al., 1990, 1992).

To say that women's emotional responses after a voluntary legal abortion are incongruent with a PTSD framework is not to say that abortion cannot be made traumatic or that it has no relationship to mental health. However, understanding the mental health of women after they have a voluntary legal abortion requires an alternative framework. In keeping with the approach of the American Psychological Association's Task Force on Postabortion Emotional Responses (Adler et al., 1990, 1992), we believe a stress and coping framework is more appropriate for conceptualizing the findings in the scientific literature.

Abortion and Mental Health: The View from the Scientific Literature

Beginning with the National Academy of Sciences (1975), every responsible scientific review has concluded that legal abortion does not have severe and long-lasting negative effects on most women, especially when the abortion occurs during the first trimester (Adler et al., 1990, 1992; Major et al., 2002; Russo, 1992, 2000; Denious & Russo, 2000; Stotland, 1992).

Such literature reviews have also shown that some women may have negative emotional responses after having an abortion, and have emphasized the importance of assessing the strength, identifying the predictors, and understanding the origins of those responses. It should be remembered that most women show a mixture of positive and negative emotions after abortion (Adler et al., 1990, 1992). However, having an emotion is not the same as having a mental disorder. A woman may check off negative emotions such as anxiety, guilt, or shame on a symptom list, but that is not sufficient to determine whether her emotional distress has clinical significance. Indeed, evidence suggests that although combinations of both positive and negative emotions are often reported, positive emotions are typically felt more strongly (Adler, 1975).

Researchers have identified a number of predictors of women's mental health after abortion. The most important is a woman's *previous* mental health. Abortion is an intensely personal decision. Its outcomes depend on the pregnancy's meaning to the woman, including whether the pregnancy was originally wanted. If a woman has difficulty in deciding to have an abortion, is uncomfortable with her decision-making process, or feels coerced into having an abortion, she is at a relatively higher risk for negative outcomes.

These factors are obviously intercorrelated and may result in delay in obtaining an abortion. Later abortions are associated with poorer mental health outcomes, possibly because they are associated with problems in the decision-making process (including learning that a wanted pregnancy has a serious fetal defect) but also because the procedure is more painful or there is a higher risk for complications. In contrast, if a woman obtains a first trimester abortion, has high expectations for being able to cope with the abortion, has social support for her decision, and good quality health care, she is at little risk for negative outcomes (Adler et al., 1990, 1992).

Identifying predictors is not the same as demonstrating a causal sequence of events. In a longitudinal study of predictors of women's well-being, Russo and Zierk (1992) found that previous positive well-being and current coping resources (more education, being employed, higher income, and fewer children) all independently predicted better postabortion well-being. Number of abortions was correlated with all of these variables, but had no independent relationship to well-being when they were controlled. That is not to say that abortion had no role in shaping these women's well-being. Insofar as having unwanted children would have detracted from their ability to pursue education, get a good job, earn a higher income, and avoid large family sizes, abortion made an indirect positive contribution to the mental health of these women and their families. That contribution was mediated through these other factors. Russo and Zierk (1992) also found that women who had experienced repeat abortions also had lower well-being than women who had experienced one abortion. This difference was primarily explained by preexisting well-being.

Later analyses of this data set (Russo & Dabul, 1997) showed that these basic findings held regardless of race (Black or White) and religion (Catholic or non-Catholic). Thus, Russo and Dabul (1997) emphasized that therapists who provide psychological services to women who have had unwanted pregnancies terminated by abortion "should explore the origins of women's mental health problems in events occurring before as well as during and after the experience . . ." (p. 29).

Obvious factors for exploration include the biological, psychological, and social factors associated with risk for poor mental health outcomes in women, including low self-esteem and feelings of hopelessness, low education and income, low instrumentality/self-efficacy, marital conflict and inequality, and effects of prejudice and discrimination based on gender, race, ethnicity, and other social categories (see McGrath, Keita, Strickland, & Russo, 1990; Russo & Green, 1993).

Childhood physical and sexual abuse and partner violence have historically been ignored despite their profound consequences for women's physical and mental health as well as their social relationships (Koss et al., 1994). Many psychological consequences of childhood abuse and intimate violence are associated with increased risk of unwanted pregnancy, including low self-esteem, depression, and feelings of alienation, dissociation, and powerlessness. Physical and sexual abuse are also linked to high-risk sexual behavior, substance abuse, earlier age at first intercourse, and earlier pregnancy (Russo and Denious, 1998b, reviewed this literature).

Partner violence has been linked to increased risk for unwanted pregnancies, whether or not such pregnancies are terminated by abortion. Among women giving birth, women whose pregnancies were unwanted and mistimed have substantially higher rates of partner violence compared to women overall (70% vs. 43%, respectively; Gazmararian et al., 1995). Russo and Denious

(2000) found that women who reported having had at least one abortion were also more likely than other women to report histories of victimization, including childhood physical abuse (26% vs.11%), sexual abuse (24% vs. 8%), rape (4% vs. 2%), and having a violent partner (23% vs. 12%). In this context, it is not surprising that some women who have a history of abortion also exhibit symptoms of post-traumatic stress and depression.

A stress and coping model provides a complex and dynamic framework for understanding how preexisting conditions and current circumstances can affect a woman's responses to a negative life event. It also conceptualizes her as an active agent who can come to control her responses to conditions she may not be responsible for and has no power to change. As Brenda Major and her colleagues (Major et al., 1998) concluded from their longitudinal research on the effectiveness of women's coping responses to abortion:

> . . . it is each woman's personal appraisals of the abortion that matter–how stressful or anxiety-provoking she regards it, and how well she expects to be able to cope with it. These appraisals are shaped, in part, by the personal resources that the woman has to draw upon, including personality attributes such as high self-esteem and perceived control, as well as the support of significant others. (p. 749)

Major et al.'s research demonstrated the crucial role that positive reframing can have in coping with unwanted pregnancy and abortion: The more women used positive reframing and acceptance to cope, the better adjusted they were on all outcome measures after the abortion, and the more satisfied they were with their decision. These findings are similar to those of research on coping of women with breast cancer (Carver et al., 1993), which showed that greater use of cognitive coping strategies was associated with lower stress. This research provides strong evidence that effective clinical intervention with women who have negative postabortion emotional responses involves helping them to use effective means of coping and to reframe their experience in a positive way.

Misinformation and Myth

> *Clearly, once a young woman is pregnant, it is no longer a choice between having a baby or not having a baby. It is a choice between having a baby or having an abortion; it is a choice between having a baby or having a traumatic experience.*

–David C. Reardon (2002)

In contrast to scientifically oriented researchers, antiabortion activists rely on anecdotal "evidence," case studies, and misinterpretation of findings to portray abortion as a mental health threat. For example, the qualitative dissertation research of Anne Speckhard (1985) has been widely cited as evidence for a "postabortion syndrome" despite the fact that it can tell us little about the normative experience of abortion patients and cannot separate the effects of abortion *per se* from the coercive, punitive social context in which it was experienced by these women. Ironically, the time between the women's retrospective accounts and their most recent abortion varied from 1 to 25 years, with both legal *and illegal* abortions included in the sample. Today about 9 of 10 women have legal abortions during the first trimester, a very different experience from having a late abortion. In Speckhard's (1985) study, 46% of the women had abortions in the second trimester; 4 percent in the third. Ironically, the horrible experiences described by the women who had illegal abortions are used to claim that early abortion under legal circumstances will have similar traumatic effects.

Antiabortion activists also misinterpret quantitative studies that compare "aborting" women to women who give birth. They claim that elevated psychological distress typically found in the former group (when preexisting conditions are not controlled) is grounds for denying women access to abortion in order to protect their mental health. They assert that abortion is a severe risk for anxiety, depression, substance abuse, and suicide, among other conditions. These interpretations require persistent dismissal of the principle that "correlation is not causation" and a dogged failure to recognize that none of a pregnant woman's alternatives–terminating the pregnancy, bearing and keeping the child, or giving the child up for adoption–are without mental health implications.

Antiabortion messages have profound mental health implications beyond the fact that they undermine women's self-efficacy for coping after abortion. On one hand, women who have abortions are stigmatized and face social ostracism. On the other, motherhood is culturally idealized, which leads pregnant women to feel ambivalent about not enthusiastically embracing all childbearing opportunities. Negative effects of unwanted childbearing for women, their families, and society, which are substantial and well documented, are blissfully ignored (David, 1992; Russo, 1992). That women can hold moral pro-choice views–such as the belief that it is immoral for a woman to bring a child into the world when she knows she cannot assume the responsibility of caring for it–goes unrecognized. In this context, even highly educated pro-choice women may be vulnerable to guilt in response to antiabortion messages that describe the decision to have an abortion as rooted in ignorance, fear, and selfishness (e.g., Elliot Institute, 1997).

Antiabortion activists emphasize adoption as the moral, "healthy" alternative for pregnant women who believe they cannot raise a child. Not considered are the potential negative psychological and social consequences of adoption to the parties involved. It is interesting that factors that predict women's negative postabortion emotional responses also predict negative postadoption responses (see Russo, 1992, for a review of this literature). Although the focus in this article is abortion issues, many of the points made here apply to all women who must deal with unwanted pregnancies however their pregnancies are resolved.

From Symptoms to Syndrome: The Dangers of Misattribution

Research on the relationship between cognitive appraisals and emotional reactions has revealed that the attribution of agency is critical for shaping emotional responses to negative life events. Attributing the cause of a negative event to circumstances results in sadness. In contrast, attributing the cause to others results in anger, contempt, and disgust (Ellsworth, 1994; Ellsworth & Smith, 1988). Most women report that their abortion is a result of their circumstances, e.g., they cannot afford a child, they are not prepared to make changes in their lives, or they are in an unstable relationship (Russo, Horn, & Schwartz, 1992; Torres & Forrest, 1988). Such women would be expected to report feeling sad after having an abortion, and indeed women do often report sadness after having an abortion (Adler et al., 1992). Although this sadness is typically transitory, it could leave women vulnerable to recruitment into "support groups" where rumination and reconstruction of the appraisal process can transform it into anger and more severe depression (Nolen-Hoeksema, 1987).

Women's cognitive appraisals of their abortion are targeted in these "support groups"; under the guise of "healing" women are encouraged to translate sadness into anger at their abortion providers. They are told that they were betrayed by their doctors; that they were denied information needed to make an informed decision; that risks of psychological and medical outcomes of abortion were hidden from them; that characteristics of the fetus were not portrayed accurately (in particular, that it experienced pain); and that they were not given the opportunity to think about alternatives (adoption, financial support). They are then encouraged to become active in the antichoice movement and to sue their physicians for not providing informed consent about emotional damage caused by abortion (see Russo and Denious, 1998a, for a description of such tactics). For example, a Website sponsored by Priests for Life asks supporters to "encourage mothers who have been harmed by abortion to bring suits against the abortion industry," and provides a list of telephone numbers of organizations that will help women bring malpractice suits (Farley, 1995).

Anne Speckhard's (1985) work described above provides a disturbing portrayal of how antiabortion groups can manipulate women's appraisals of their abortion experience:

> In these social systems [prolife and fundamental religious groups] subjects found members who allowed them to freely discuss their feelings of grief, guilt, loneliness, anger, and despair . . . members of these systems were not adverse to discussing the details of the abortion experience with

particular reference to concern over pain that the fetus may have experienced and damage that may have occurred to the subjects' reproductive organs. (pp. 139-140)

Her words show how such groups can lay a foundation for recruiting women to file malpractice suits and how their misinformation about fetal development is a particular source of distress:

They became increasingly angry about the way abortion had been explained to them. . . . Many learned a great deal from prolife groups about fetal development which initially increased their guilt, grief, and anger. (pp. 140-141)

Given that antiabortion messages are designed to manipulate women's appraisal process and to link their psychological distress to the abortion, misattribution of symptoms that result from previous or concurrent experiences is of grave concern. Anxious and depressed women seeking support are prey for individuals who can capitalize on the fact that abortion is a concrete and specific event that can function as a "lightning rod" for highly charged negative emotions that may be related to a woman's body and sexuality, her functioning as a wife, mother, or intimate partner, and her beliefs about her right to put her needs over those of others (Lemkau, 1988). Given the correlation between a history of victimization and unintended pregnancy, symptoms of post-traumatic stress from exposure to intimate violence are at risk for misattribution (Russo & Denious, 1998b, 2000).

People do continually reconstruct and reinterpret past events in the light of subsequent experiences. Under stressful and tragic circumstances, ideas of punishment and retribution can surface. Stressful conditions such as infertility, infant death, or catastrophic illness thus are often characterized by depressed mood and cognitive distortions. In such circumstances, women may come to link their negative feelings to an earlier abortion as well as other events in their life history, particularly when there is an intensive campaign to construct such linkages. We do not argue that these *post hoc* reconstructions are unimportant or that women's concerns should be trivialized. We are not saying that all of the symptoms found in every woman are due to preexisting conditions. Our point is that such connections and their associated feelings should be examined in therapy with a licensed mental health professional who does not prejudge their underlying causality and who explores the dynamics of their origins beyond the abortion experience.

In true Orwellian fashion, antiabortion activists misrepresent concerns about misattribution of symptoms that originate from preexisting conditions as "blaming the victim" for her negative responses to abortion. The point that prejudgment is the concern and that negative emotions may be due to preexisting conditions and thus would be present even if the women had chosen to have a child is not addressed. Researchers are portrayed as arguing that "if women were tougher, they wouldn't be so upset over having an abortion" and as being unsympathetic to women's problems. Given the history of silence around violence issues, attempts to distract women from exploring effects of preexisting conditions and to manipulate women's causal attributions of PTSD symptoms to advance a political agenda are simply reprehensible.

APPROACHES, ISSUES, AND RESOURCES IN THERAPY

Given this political context, an effective therapist needs to be knowledgeable about the literature on the physical and psychological risks associated with abortion, its precursors, and its alternatives; about fetal characteristics; and about the pros and cons of the alternatives open to abortion patients (Russo, 1992, 2000). We begin this section with a discussion of approaches therapists can use to enhance women's strategies for coping with abortion. Next, we discuss specific issues and useful techniques for working with women who have abortion concerns. Finally, we provide a brief list of resources for therapists and clients who want to know more about abortion concerns and women's issues.

Enhancing Coping Strategies

Coping strategies can determine whether having an abortion is appraised as a temporary stressor or viewed as a continuing trauma. In particular, a woman's social support, self-efficacy for coping, and methods of coping with an abortion can shape her emotional responses.

Support and validation. In a political context designed to foster shame and guilt, social support, validation, and appraisal issues become particularly important. Therapists need to address negative mental health outcomes that result from social ostracism and harassment of abortion patients (Adler, 1975; Cozzarelli & Major, 1998). Ostracism and harassment can subvert mental health by inducing negative socially based emotions, undermining social support, and encouraging unplanned and unwanted childbearing (Russo, 1992). Providing women with accurate, balanced information in a supportive setting can enhance women's sense of self-efficacy and control and help counter these effects.

Social conflict and social support from close others are significantly related to women's postabortion adjustment. Therapists should explore whether clients have or had support from others through the decision-making process and afterward. For clients experiencing particular distress, therapists should explore the possibility of coercion in the decision-making process, which is associated with more negative postabortion reactions (Adler et al., 1990, 1992; Lemkau, 1988). In their study of married abortion patients, Russo and Pope

(1993) found that women who had violent husbands were more likely to ... having made the decision to have an abortion on their own. This suggests that abused women in particular may benefit from social support interventions.

In a longitudinal study of first-trimester abortion patients, Brenda Major and her colleagues (Major et al., 1998) found that coping with abortion-related emotions through positive reframing and instrumental or emotional support-seeking was associated with lower levels of distress postabortion. In contrast, coping through venting was related to poorer adjustment, after controlling for initial distress. This finding suggests that therapists must be mindful that not all coping strategies are equally helpful. For example, support groups that foster venting and rumination rather than emotional processing and moving on from the experience may do more harm than good (Nolen-Hoeksema, 1987).

Fostering alternative appraisals and positive images. Clients may benefit from empowering books and stories, such as Patricia Lunneborg's (1992) *Abortion: A Positive Decision* or Angela Bonavoglia's (2001) *The Choices We Made*, which include positive stories of women who have coped with abortion. These books break the silence surrounding abortion, help women understand that they are not alone, and promote more optimistic appraisals of their decision and their future. Pro-choice Websites, such as HeartsSite.com and peaceafterabortion.com, which are devoted to providing healing alternatives to the negative images of abortion found in cyberspace, can also help in showing how different women have dealt with issues that troubled them after abortion.

Self-efficacy. Research suggests that perceived social support from family, friends, and partners is related to higher self-efficacy for coping with abortion, which, in turn, is related to better postabortion adjustment (Major et al., 1990). Therapists can assess clients' perceived self-efficacy for coping with abortion and use therapeutic interventions to enhance clients' self-efficacy for coping in general and with the particular circumstances, i.e., intra- or interpersonal, financial, cultural issues. These approaches are particularly congruent with feminist therapy goals of increasing women's awareness of how the sociopolitical context contributes to women's distress (e.g., the political context of abortion) and empowering women to reclaim influence over their circumstances.

Issues and Strategies in Therapy

Given the current political context, what can a therapist do to provide effective, empowering, and ethical treatment of clients? Basic principles of practice apply when doing therapy with women dealing with abortion-related concerns, but therapists also need to be aware of unique concerns and special challenges when dealing with abortion issues, and informed about specific resources for dealing with them.

Avoiding prejudgment. Therapists should avoid prejudging the causes of their clients' distress. Although women from all walks of life experience unwanted pregnancy, it occurs most often among women already facing stressful life circumstances (e.g., poverty, discrimination, physical and sexual abuse). Stress of an unwanted pregnancy not only exacerbates women's risk of developing mental health problems, but also increases susceptibility to the myths and misinformation spread by antiabortion activists who prey on women's vulnerabilities. When therapists are mindful of potential ways women's attributions of distress may be manipulated, they can help clients better determine the origins of their distress. Women who decide to have an abortion typically experience a combination of positive and negative emotions, including ambivalence, sadness, and distress. Strength and duration of negative emotions vary significantly, depending on a woman's values and life circumstances. Most often, negative reactions are temporary and a "normal" part of what, for some women, involves a process of grieving for what might have been.

As Freeman (1978) has observed, the choice of whether to bear a child may be the first time a woman has had to make a truly important decision. Unwanted pregnancy forces a woman to confront her values as well as the realities of her life. This process involves painful self-judgments and a loss of illusions. Antiabortion efforts to construct a "postabortion syndrome" disrupt the therapeutic process by focusing the woman on the baby that might have been and pathologizing her feelings of sadness and loss. But issues of loss that need be explored in therapy are broader–indeed they may encompass a host of discrepancies in a woman's vision of herself as a caring and moral person, in her relationship to her husband or intimate partner, and in her identity as a mother, among others (for some examples of the complexities underlying negative feelings in response to abortion see Torre-Bueno, 1996, or visit www.peaceafterabortion.com). Effective therapists recognize that feelings of ambivalence, sadness, and regret are normal after making such a momentous decision and help the client put those feelings into context. They avoid pathologizing the process of recovery, and carefully attend to the unique experiences and histories of each individual client.

Certainly, some women experience distress about their decision to have an abortion, particularly when they have been coerced by others (e.g., a partner or parent), and/or when they have experienced trauma from the procedure because it was performed in an improper setting due to legal or practical restrictions. However, for the majority of clients, the greatest distress is caused by the circumstances surrounding the abortion, such as a partner that was unsupportive, an economic situation, or fears based on misinformation, such as a fear of developing breast cancer or being unable to bear future children. Helping women to understand the multiple causes of their distress, rather than pinning all negative emotions on the abortion itself, will help empower them to take control of their life circumstances.

Therapists may invite clients to examine the positive aspects of the abortion decision, including feelings of relief or control over her fate. To the extent that women have internalized cultural messages that abortion is a selfish choice, they may not be able to recognize the caring and responsibility of their decision, and may even feel guilty about the positive emotions associated with the decision to terminate an unwanted pregnancy. Ironically, the cultural context is such that women who have little ambivalence about their decision feel guilty about not feeling guilty, and therapists must address those issues as well.

Constructions of the Fetus

To My Baby

Although now is not the time, I know your spirit (your soul) is meant for me. They say that we all love rest and sleep, so may you rest your soul a little longer. The body is just a rented car for the soul. Although when I get my chance to bring you back you will have a different body, I know the soul that is meant for me is in there. I love you! Until then, forget me not.

–Anonymous (HeartsSite.com, n.d.)

Therapists must equip women to recognize how images of the fetus are manipulated to create feelings of distress and guilt in women. Women are told that because their "babies" did not experience the "testing grounds" of earthly existence, they are doomed to limbo and denied access to heaven. Alternative views such as the one expressed above that appears on the HeartsSite Website are not recognized in such messages.

In addition to exposing women to alternative viewpoints, therapists need to be prepared to explain how the nervous system develops and what this means for the idea that the fetus can feel pain. Very few women have abortions during the last trimester of pregnancy, but their lack of knowledge of fetal development can make the idea that their embryo or fetus might have felt pain very troubling. Practitioners can reassure women by giving them accurate information, including the fact that the neocortex, where human consciousness, thinking, problem-solving, and language are located, does not develop until late in pregnancy, in the third trimester. Before that part of the brain develops and is neurally connected with the rest of the developing fetal body, the idea that a fetus can "think" or "feel pain" has no basis in biological fact (Flowers, 1992). Misrepresentation of fetal development is a powerful strategy whose influence goes beyond cognitive effects. Antiabortion protesters and antiabortion Websites present images of developed (often third trimester or stillborn) fetuses, and through repeated pairings, clients may come to associate those images with their abortion experience. Through classical conditioning, vulnerable women may become traumatized by these images, and even men and women who have never had an abortion may be conditioned to feel uncomfortable with the topic. To counter such effects, therapists can educate women about fetal de-

., and, if necessary and appropriate, do "exposure therapy" by provid-
:tive images, pictures, or videotapes to clients.

Cultural Sensitivity

*For us, as African-American women who came up through slavery and
were forced to breed, we can't ever give away the opportunity to make
those decisions for ourselves.*

–Byllye Avery (2001, p. 154)

Cultural sensitivity is always important in therapy, and the issue of abortion
may require specific sensitivities because moral and religious values intersect
with identities conferred by race, class, or ethnicity. At the same time that historical linkages between coercive abortion and eugenics movements may have led
some poor women and Women of Color to feel ambivalence on the issue of
abortion, they have also heightened commitment to reproductive choice, particularly for women whose choices have been limited due to racist and classist poli-
cies and practices (Avery, 2001; Roberts, 1990; Wyatt, 1997). Therapists need
to be knowledgeable about the diversity of religious and cultural beliefs about
abortion (see Maguire, 2001). They also need to understand the heterogeneity of
beliefs among individuals and within religious cultural groups, which is represented, for example, by groups such as Catholics for a Free Choice.
Some women may have chosen abortion despite holding beliefs that abortion is wrong. In such situations, therapists should help women cope with the
conflicting emotions they may experience. When counseling religious women
conflicted between abortion and their spiritual beliefs, therapists may help
them remember their God's or spiritual leader's capacity for forgiveness
(Fisher, Castle, & Garrity, 1998; Torre-Bueno, 1996).

Promoting positive sexual health. Improving women's emotional and physical health requires addressing sexual health, including a client's beliefs about
contraception, which (if any) methods she uses, and barriers to contraceptive
use. Concern about sexual health is particularly important for women who
have experienced an unwanted pregnancy, as they are likely to have become
pregnant due to obstacles or struggles related to these issues. Circumstances
that place women at risk for unwanted pregnancy–including men's control of
sexual decision making, men's violence against women, and poverty–also
place women at greater risk for contracting HIV and other sexually transmitted
diseases. If appropriate, therapists should help clients develop a plan for effective pregnancy and disease prevention. Fisher et al. (1998) have suggested using "non-directive *if-then* statements," such as "*if* you don't want to get
pregnant, *then* it is important to take your pill everyday" (p. 320, emphasis in
original), which are logical, nonjudgmental, and ultimately empower the client
to make her own decision, an important principle of feminist praxis.

Religion

RESOURCES

Given the extensive dissemination of inaccurate information about abortion, psychotherapists have an ethical mandate to inform themselves about these issues. Space limitations preclude a full exploration of the complex and profound issues women face when dealing with unwanted pregnancy. In addition to the material cited above which is found in the reference list, here are added resources to help with specific issues.

Psychological Issues

The Society for the Psychology of Women (Division 35 of the American Psychological Association) sponsors a new Website under the aegis of the ProChoice Forum designed to counter myths related to abortion and to increase research-based knowledge and informed opinion about psychological aspects of abortion and related reproductive health issues. In the Practice Issues section contributors discuss issues and best practices for abortion counseling, psychotherapy, and other mental health service delivery. It also provides links to other relevant sites <http://www.prochoiceforum.org.uk/>.

Religion

Religious Coalition for Reproductive Choice: <http://www.rcrc.org/>.
Spiritual comfort: Before and after an abortion by Anne Baker and Rev. Annie P. Clark: <http://www.hopeclinic.com/publications.htm>.
Catholics for a Free Choice: <http://www.cath4choice.org>.

General Resources and Support

Brick, P., & Taverner, B. (2001). *Educating about abortion.* Hackensack, NJ: Planned Parenthood of Greater Northern New Jersey. This manual explores abortion issues in a series of chapters that contain well-defined objectives, hand-outs, and activities.
Kaufman, K. (1997). *The abortion resource handbook.* New York: Fireside.

Challenging Myths

For general information see:

The Alan Guttmacher Institute provides online access to its journals as well as a host of fact sheets and reports related to reproductive health: <http://www.agi-sa.org/>.

For information on the relationship of abortion to breast cancer, see: <http://www.cancer.org/eprise/main/docroot/CRI/content/CRI_2_6x_Can_Having_ an_ Abortion_Cause_or_Contribute_to_Breast_Cancer?>.

National Cancer Institute. (1999). Cancer Facts: Abortion and Breast Cancer [Online]. <http://cis.nci.nih.gov/fCact/3_53.htm>.

Some Accessible Readings with Broader Coverage of Related Issues

Bem, L. (1993). *The lenses of gender: Transforming the debate about sexual equality.* New Haven, CT: Yale University Press.

Chrisler, J. C., Golden, C., & Rozee, P. (Eds.). (2004). *Lectures on the psychology of women* (3rd ed.). New York: McGraw-Hill.

Steil, J. (1997). *Marital equality: Its relationship to the well-being of husbands and wives.* Thousand Oaks, CA: Sage.

Ussher, J. (2000). *Women's health: Contemporary international perspectives.* London: British Psychological Society.

Wyatt, G. E. (1997). *Stolen women: Reclaiming our sexuality, taking back our lives.* New York: Wiley.

CONCLUSION

The substantial body of data that suggests that having a legal abortion is not a negative factor with regard to mental health for most women is encouraging (Adler et al., 1990, 1992; Russo, 1992). Abortion-related stress typically does not exceed women's coping resources, and, in any case, having an unwanted child is not a stress-free alternative, so a one-sided concern with abortion's mental health effects distorts a complex picture. Some women are indeed troubled by having had an abortion, and therapists should be sensitive and responsive to their concerns. Nonetheless, there is no evidence for widespread, severe, or long-lasting effects of legal abortion, particularly in the first trimester when most women have abortions.

The campaign to construct a "postabortion syndrome" has the potential to change this situation, however, particularly if the misinformation spread by antiabortion activists succeeds in manipulating women's appraisals, undermining their feelings of self-efficacy for coping with an abortion, deterring social support, fostering shame and guilt, and ultimately achieving the end of making abortion illegal. Further, unwanted pregnancy and abortion are correlated with preexisting conditions and life circumstances–including childhood physical and sexual abuse, rape, and battering–that have a history of being ignored by mainstream or traditional therapists. Insofar as the well documented, profound, and long-lasting effects on mental health of these traumatic events are misattributed to having an abortion, the underlying issues will not be addressed and women's mental health will be ill-served. By being informed about antiabortion messages that undermine mental health, all therapists can provide more effective therapy and better serve their clients.

REFERENCES

(Qualitative material and other resources for therapy are asterisked.)

Adler, N. E. (1975). Emotional responses of women following therapeutic abortion. *American Journal of Orthopsychiatry, 45,* 446-454.

Adler, N. E., David, H. P., Major, B., Roth, S., Russo, N. F., & Wyatt, G. (1990). Psychological responses after abortion. *Science, 248,* 41-44.

Adler, N. E., David, H., Major, B., Roth, S., Russo, N., & Wyatt, G. (1992). Psychological factors in abortion: A review. *American Psychologist, 47,* 1194-1204.

Alan Guttmacher Institute (2002). *Induced abortion: Facts in brief.* New York: Alan Guttmacher Institute.

*Avery, B. (2001). Byllye Avery. In A. Bonavoglia (Ed.), *The choices we made: Twenty-five women and men speak out about abortion* (pp. 147-154). New York: Four Walls Eight Windows.

*Bonavoglia, A. (Ed.). (2001). *The choices we made: Twenty-five women and men speak out about abortion.* New York: Four Walls Eight Windows.

Carver, C. S., Pozo, C., Harris, S. D., Noriega, V., Scheier, M. F., Robinson, D. S., Ketcham, A., Moffat, F. L., & Clark, K. C. (1993). How coping mediates the effect of optimism on distress: A study of women with early stage breast cancer. *Journal of Personality and Social Psychology, 65,* 375-390.

Cozzarelli, C., & Major, B. (1998). The impact of antiabortion activities on women seeking abortions. In L. J. Beckman & S. M. Harvey (Eds.), *The new civil war: The psychology, culture, and politics of abortion* (pp. 81-104). Washington, DC: American Psychological Association.

David, H. P. (1985). Post-abortion and post-partum psychiatric hospitalization. *CIBA Foundation Symposium, 115,* 150-164.

David, H. P. (1992). Born unwanted: Long-term developmental effects of denied abortion. *Journal of Social Issues, 48,* 163-181.

David, H. P., Dytrych, Z., Matejcek, Z., & Schüller, V. (Eds.). (1988). *Born unwanted: Developmental effects of denied abortion.* New York: Springer.

Denious, J., & Russo, N. F. (2000). The socio-political context of abortion and its relationship to women's mental health. In J. Ussher (Ed.), *Women's health: Contempo rary international perspectives* (pp. 431-439). London: British Psychological Society.

Elliot Institute (1997). *Let Us Show You How We Will STOP ABORTION.* Advertising flyer, Elliot Institute, P. O. Box 7348, Springfield, IL, USA.

Ellsworth, P. C. (1994). Sense, culture, and sensibility. In S. Kitayama & H. R. Markus (Eds.), *Emotion and culture: Empirical studies of mutual influence* (pp. 23-50). Washington, DC: American Psychological Association.

Ellsworth, P. C., & Smith, C. A. (1988). From appraisal to emotion: Differences among unpleasant feelings. *Motivation and Emotion, 12,* 271-302.

Farley, C. (1995, Mar. 13). Malpractice as a weapon. *Time, 145,* p. 65.

*Fisher, B., Castle, M. A., & Garrity, J. M. (1998). A cognitive approach to patient-centered abortion care. In L. J. Beckman & S. M. Harvey (Eds.), *The new civil war: The psychology, culture, and politics of abortion* (pp. 301-328). Washington, DC: American Psychological Association.

*Flowers, M. J. (1992). Coming into being: The prenatal development of humans. In J. D. Butler & D. F. Walbert (Eds.), *Abortion, medicine, and the law* (4th ed., pp. 437-452). New York: Facts on File.

Freeman, E. W. (1978). Abortion: Subjective attitudes and feelings. *Family Planning Perspectives, 10,* 150-155.

Gazmararian, J. A., Adams, M. M., Saltzman, L. E., Johnson, C. H., Bruce, F. C., Marks, J. S., & Zahniser, S. C. (1995). The relationship between pregnancy intendedness and physical violence in mothers of newborns. *Obstetrics & Gynecology, 85,* 1031-1038.

*Johnston, P. (1998). Pregnant? Need help? Pregnancy options workbook. This excellent resource is available online: <http://www.ferre.org/workbook/index.html>. Order from: Ferre Institute, 124 Front St., Binghamton, NY 13905. FAX (607) 724-8290.

*Kahn-Edrington, M. (1979). Abortion counseling. *Counseling Psychologist, 8,* 37-38.

Koss, M. P., Goodman, L. A., Browne, A., Fitzgerald, L., Keita, G. P., & Russo, N. F. (1994). *No safe haven: Male violence against women at home, at work, and in the community.* Washington, DC: American Psychological Association.

*Kushner, E. (1997). *Experiencing abortion: A weaving of women's words.* Binghamton, NY: The Haworth Press, Inc.

Lazarus, R., & Folkman, S. (1984). *Stress, appraisal, and coping.* New York: Springer.

*Lemkau, J. P. (1988). Emotional sequelae of abortion: Implications for clinical practice. *Psychology of Women Quarterly, 12,* 461-472.

*Lunneborg, P. (1992). *Abortion: A positive decision.* New York: Bergin & Garvey.

*Maguire, D. C. (2001). *Sacred choices: The right to contraception and abortion in ten world religions.* Minneapolis, MN: Fortress Press.

Major, B., & Cozzarelli, C. (2000). Abortion. In A. E. Kazdin (Ed.), *Encyclopedia of psychology* (vol. 1, pp. 1-5). London: Oxford University Press.

Major, B., Cozzarelli, C., Sciacchitano, A. M., Cooper, M. L., Testa, M., & Mueller, P. M. (1990). Perceived social support, self-efficacy, and adjustment to abortion. *Journal of Personality and Social Psychology, 59,* 452-463.

Major, B., Richards, C., Cooper, M. L., Cozzarelli, C., & Zubek, J. (1998). Personal resilience, cognitive appraisals, and coping: An integrative model of adjustment to abortion. *Journal of Personality and Social Psychology, 74,* 735-752.

Major, B., Zubek, J. M., Cooper, M. L., Cozzarelli, C., & Richards, C. (1997). Mixed messages: Implications of social conflict and social support within close relationships for adjustment to a stressful life event. *Journal of Personality and Social Psychology, 72,* 1349-1363.

McGrath, E., Keita, G. P., Strickland, B. R., & Russo, N. F. (Eds.). (1990). *Women and depression: Risk factors and treatment issues.* Washington, DC: American Psychological Association.

National Academy of Sciences (1975). *Legalized abortion and the public health.* Washington DC: National Academy Press.

Nolen-Hoeksema, S. (1987). *Sex differences in depression.* Stanford, CA: Stanford University Press.

Reardon, D. C. (2002). *A new strategy for ending abortion: Learning the truth–Telling the truth.* Website: <http://www.afterabortion.org>.

Roberts, D. E. (1990). The future of reproductive choice for poor women and women of color. *Women's Right Law Reporter, 12,* 59-67.

Roe v. Wade. 410 U.S. 113 (1973).

Russo, N. F. (1992). Psychological aspects of unwanted pregnancy and its resolution. In J. D. Butler & D. F. Walbert (Eds.), *Abortion, medicine and the law* (4th ed., pp. 593-626). New York: Facts on File.

Russo, N. F. (2000). Understanding emotional responses after abortion. In J. C. Chrisler, C. Golden, & P. Rozee (Eds.), *Lectures on the psychology of women* (2nd ed.) (pp. 260-273). New York: McGraw-Hill.

Russo, N. F., & Dabul, A. (1997). The relationship of abortion to well-being: Do race and religion make a difference? *Professional Psychology: Research and Practice, 28,* 23-31.

Russo, N. F., & Denious, J. (1998a). Why is abortion such a controversial issue in the United States? In L. J. Beckman & S. M. Harvey (Eds.), *The new civil war: The psychology, culture, and politics of abortion* (pp. 25-60). Washington, DC: American Psychological Association.

Russo, N. F., & Denious, J. (1998b). Understanding the relationship of violence against women to unwanted pregnancy and its resolution. In L. J. Beckman & S. M. Harvey (Eds.), *The new civil war: The psychology, culture, and politics of abortion* (pp. 211-234). Washington, DC: American Psychological Association.

Russo, N. F., & Denious, J. E. (2001). Violence in the lives of women having abortions: Implications for public policy and practice. *Professional Psychology: Research and Practice, 32,* 142-150

Russo, N. F., Denious, J., Keita, G. P., & Koss, M. P. (1997). Intimate violence and black women's health. *Women's Health: Research on Gender, Behavior, and Public Policy, 3,* 315-348.

Russo, N. F., & Green, B. L. (1993). Women and mental health. In F. L. Denmark & M. A. Paludi (Eds.), *Psychology of women: A handbook of issues and theories* (pp. 379-436). Westport, CT: Greenwood Press.

Russo, N. F., Horn, J., & Schwartz, R. (1992). U.S. abortion in context: Selected characteristics and motivations of women seeking abortion. *Journal of Social Issues, 48,* 182-201.

Russo, N. F., & Pope, L. (1993, May). *Implications of violence against women for reproductive health: Focus on abortion services.* Paper presented at the Conference on Psychology and Women's Health: Creating a Psychosocial Agenda for the 21st Century, Washington, DC.

Russo, N. F., & Zierk, K. (1992). Abortion, childbearing, and women's well-being. *Professional Psychology: Research and Practice, 23,* 269-280.

Solinger, R. (Ed.). (1998). *Abortion wars: A half century of struggle, 1950-2000.* Berkeley, CA: University of California Press.

Speckhard, A. C. (1985). *The psycho-social aspects of stress following an abortion.* Unpublished doctoral dissertation, University of Minnesota.

Stotland, N. (1992). The myth of the abortion trauma syndrome. *Journal of the American Medical Association, 268,* 2078-2079.

*Torre-Bueno, A. (1996). *Peace after abortion.* San Diego: Pimpernel Press.

Torres, A., & Forrest, J. D. (1988). Why do women have abortions? *Family Planning Perspectives, 20*(4), 169-176.

Wilmoth, G. H., de Alteriis, M., & Bussell, D. (1992). Prevalence of psychological risks following legal abortion in the U.S.: Limits of the evidence. *Journal of Social Issues, 48,* 37-60.

*Wyatt, G. E. (1997). *Stolen women: Reclaiming our sexuality, taking back our lives.* New York: John Wiley & Sons.

Psychological Issues and Interventions
with Infertile Patients

Ann Rosen Spector

SUMMARY. Of the estimated 10-15 percent of American couples who are infertile, approximately 50 percent will never bear children. Those who consult a psychotherapist have a wide range of both pragmatic and emotional needs. Psychotherapists can help women, men, and couples [gay or straight, married or unmarried] cope with infertility and sterility, as a transitory or permanent state. In this article I discuss issues relative to the marriage/relationship, sexual behavior and identity, exploration of outcome alternatives, parenting concerns, and the depression and anxiety that generally result from reproductive failure. *[Article copies available for a fee from The Haworth Document Delivery Service: 1-800-HAWORTH. E-mail address: <docdelivery@haworthpress.com> Website: <http://www.HaworthPress. com> © 2004 by The Haworth Press, Inc. All rights reserved.]*

KEYWORDS. Infertility, marital relationships, sexual relations, motherhood role, childlessness, parenthood

Ann Rosen Spector, PhD, is a clinical psychologist in private practice in Philadelphia, Pennsylvania, with a specialty in couples' therapy and health issues, including infertility. She is also an adjunct faculty member of the Department of Psychology, Rutgers University, Camden, New Jersey.

Address correspondence to: Ann Rosen Spector, 1508 Medical Tower Building, 255 S. 17th Street, Philadelphia, PA 19103-6215 (E-mail: ARSPECTO@camden.rutgers.edu).

The author is enormously grateful for the editorial and emotional support of her good friend and mentor, Janet Golden.

[Haworth co-indexing entry note]: "Psychological Issues and Interventions with Infertile Patients." Spector, Ann Rosen. Co-published simultaneously in *Women & Therapy* (The Haworth Press, Inc.) Vol. 27, No. 3/4, 2004, pp. 91-105; and: *From Menarche to Menopause: The Female Body in Feminist Therapy* (ed: Joan C. Chrisler) The Haworth Press, Inc., 2004, pp. 91-105. Single or multiple copies of this article are available for a fee from The Haworth Document Delivery Service [1-800-HAWORTH, 9:00 a.m. - 5:00 p.m. (EST). E-mail address: docdelivery@haworthpress.com].

10.1300/J015v27n03_07

Most societies are pronatalist, and most women want to be mothers (Spector, 1985). Historically, this was to ensure the survival of the group. Given current world overpopulation and the development of the modern family, such concerns may be anachronistic (Polit, 1978). Indeed, young women today, married or not, are more likely to focus on issues of abortion, contraception, and delaying childbirth. Despite the transition from high to low fertility and new family ideals, most people still expect to have children; more important: they expect to be *able* to have children.

Infertility has typically been presumed to be a woman's problem, and the "barren" woman is a more culturally salient figure than the sterile or impotent man because it is the woman who bears or fails to bear children. In addition, women are presumed to have a maternal instinct and a biological clock that impel them to want to be mothers. The mother role has been central to the lives of most adult women (Bernard, 1974; Poston & Kramer, 1980; Russo, 1979) and, historically and traditionally, to fail to assume this role has raised questions about one's adult status and one's femininity.

Prior to the Civil War, infertility was largely defined as a moral dilemma, and the remedy was to be found in prayer, piety, and consultation with religious leaders. With the rise of the medical profession (and obstetrics and gynecology as a specialty), infertility came to be seen as a physical problem that requires medical intervention (Marsh, 1997; Rosenberg & Smith-Rosenberg, 1976). This view remains in place today.

Despite the long history of individual struggles with the problem of infertility, it is only in the last few decades that childlessness, both voluntary and involuntary, has received much attention in the popular press or scholarly literature (Poston & Kramer, 1980). Perhaps this lack of attention reflected social disapproval of childlessness as well as the invisibility that "victims" sought for reasons of privacy. Alternatively, it may have reflected a perception that childlessness was not a problem. In 1966 some social scientists declared voluntary childlessness "extinct"; this notion may have derived from a misinterpretation of the demographic bulge known as the "baby boom" (Whelpton, Campbell, & Patterson, 1966). Until the 1970s, the United States did not include questions about childlessness on the census form, a further sign that it was not perceived to be a significant social issue (Mosher & Pratt, 1982).

Nevertheless, infertility is a significant problem for every person who would like to have children and cannot. The ways in which people manage infertility, in medical and psychological terms, depends to a great extent on the cultural climate in which they reside as well as the resources available to them. Support from a therapist is among the chief critical resources.

MARITAL RELATIONSHIPS

Some individuals and couples seek out psychological help when they anticipate or are experiencing delays or difficulties in achieving or sustaining a pregnancy. [Unmarried women, lesbian couples, and heterosexual cohabitators may all perceive themselves as infertile and seek treatment. For simplicity's sake, I refer to them all as couples.] The members of the couple may be at different stages of readiness to become parents, have different responses to the diagnosis and treatment of infertility, and feel more or less isolated from family and friends. One or both members of the couple may feel shame, depression, anxiety, blamed (or a need to blame), and fear of abandonment by the fertile spouse.

These issues will come up in first marriages, and are often even more pronounced in remarriages, where one spouse is already a parent.

> A male patient had three children by his early 30s. When the marriage ended, he moved more than 1,000 miles away and saw his children infrequently. Ten years later he married a successful career woman who seemed to share his preference for the largely childless lifestyle. Then they relocated back to his original city, spent a lot more time with his adolescent children, and she turned 39 . . . and she wanted to have a baby. He did not want more children, but he loved her and did not want to deny her the opportunity to become a mother. When she was unable to conceive, he was privately relieved. He was ambivalent about pursuing infertility evaluations and treatments, but he did not want to damage his marriage.

What this case illustrates is a common problem for couples: one person wants the pregnancy and child more than the other does, and communication about sensitive topics is flawed. At a time when the couple needs to be closer than ever, secrets and desires are a point of division. Wives are typically the driving force to get spouses and medical personnel to recognize that there is a problem that needs attention; they are more likely to reject the "relax and let it happen" strategy (Edelmann & Connolly, 2000; Freeman, Boxer, Rickels, Turek, & Mastrioanni, 1985; Griel, 1991; Unruh & McGrath, 1985).

The therapist's responses will depend on the format she is using and whether she is seeing the individuals separately in addition to conjoint therapy. If she is having individual sessions, she may well be aware that what one person is experiencing is not being articulated to the spouse. The goal at this point is to have each person resolve whatever issues are extant and then process the information appropriately with each other. The goal is not only to achieve a pregnancy, or to mourn the inability to do so, but also to support and strengthen the couple's relationship. If the therapist is only seeing one member of the couple, or only the couple together, she will likely be limited by selective information, either conscious or unconscious, and by biases and omissions.

Confounding the physical, sexual, and emotional difficulties are the financial hardships imposed by infertility. Most health care insurers do not cover either infertility evaluation or treatment because being childless is seen as a lifestyle "choice" issue, not a health issue. This is despite the fact that insurers reimburse for Viagra, a drug for erectile dysfunction. Therapists should be attuned to the anger this is likely to provoke among women infertility patients.

In order for medical subspecialty practices to survive and thrive, they need a substantial population to utilize their services. As a result, urban and suburban residents have more access to infertility specialists than those in rural areas, and those with greater income will also have greater access to such care. This is true both in the United States and in the United Kingdom (Doyal, 1987). If the woman or couple decide to seek psychological help, that is an added expense, which may be another source of tension for the couple. If the couple has different views regarding this expense, and different perspectives about infertility, such as how much to spend and how long to pursue treatment, then conflict is likely to emerge from decision-making *about* the infertility and therapeutic options.

In addition, medical staff may desire a different pace (either slower or quicker) for tests and treatments than the individual or couple can tolerate psychologically or afford financially. The therapist can help the patient(s) understand and evaluate the pace . . . and a need for pauses . . . and stop points . . . that are right for them, and help them negotiate with their physicians and partners regarding these decisions.

SEXUAL RELATIONS

For most couples, sexual relations are both a by-product of the intense emotional commitment as well as a physical desire and manifestation of the libido. For infertile couples, sex becomes an item on the "to do" list for achieving a pregnancy, and the strain of scheduling intercourse on demand is often one of the major stressors of the infertility experience.

> We were "saving up sperm" to have tests and "saving up sperm" to try to make a baby. It became incredibly precious fluid to us. I used to think how awful it would be if after abstaining for four days my husband had a wet dream and all was lost. (Menning, 1977, p. 108)

In other instances, there are transient bouts of impotence and concomitant performance anxiety, which can lead to increased erectile or ejaculatory dysfunction, which tends to lead to more of the same. The result can be a sense of failure for the man for impotence and for the woman for being unable to achieve a pregnancy easily｜Women, too, can believe that their sexual behavior is an impediment to fertility. Some women erroneously assume that being unable to achieve an orgasm precludes fertilization, or that too frequent or too vigorous sex leads to miscarriage. The therapist, often in conjunction with the reproductive endocrinologist, can furnish accurate information and allay these fears.

The therapist's goal is to help the couple distinguish between sex for procreation and sex for recreation and work together to make both kinds of experiences enjoyable, if only for the potential comedic value. One couple, trying to conceive during the World Series, chose the "seventh inning stretch" as the time to have intercourse; as they undressed, the wife yelled, "Play ball." They became pregnant during that cycle!

Once a couple has achieved a pregnancy or birth . . . or stopped trying, it is very important to help them reestablish a normal, loving sex life. Having had sex to achieve the goal of "baby," it is now necessary to learn again how to have sexual relations for all of the reasons that lovers have sex.

BODY IMAGE

Reproductive failure often makes people feel defective–sick when they thought all along that they were healthy. We assume throughout our lives that we will be able to have children whenever we want to do so. Most Americans spend a great deal of time, effort, and money to limit fertility by contraception or abortion. It is all the more injurious to one's sense of well-being to be unable to do what everyone else seems to do so effortlessly . . . even thoughtlessly and accidentally. Although infertile people look normal on the outside, they often feel completely abnormal about their internal selves, as manifested by imperfect reproductive capacity and performance.

The sense of a flawed body may extend to dissatisfaction with physical appearance and a heightened sense of morbidity. From childhood on, people develop not only a sense of how their bodies look and perform to themselves, but also how they think others perceive them. Infertility will pose a greater threat to self in those who have not developed a strong sense of self and body image. Infertile people will often "wear" the defect as if it is observable to others (Menning, 1997).

How can one be pretty or good-looking if all the feminine parts of the body are not there or are not in good working order? Therapists can help readjust patients' sense of normalcy and help distinguish between form and function. The sense of impairment affects not only the sense of being 100 percent woman or man, but also the sense of being a competent spouse and sexual partner. It is a contagion of defect. As one woman said about being sexually active with her spouse, "In part, it was because of my new feelings of defectiveness . . . [that I felt] 'Why bother? What for?'" (Menning, 1977, p. 130). For single women, it can extend to such sex inappropriateness as to preclude marriage; if one cannot marry and have children, then why marry? And what man would choose her, as a sexual partner or a wife (Williams & Power, 1977)?

If women see motherhood as a natural and essential part of womanhood as Freud, Deutsch, and Benedek have claimed (as cited in Allison, 1979), their resulting feelings will differ markedly from those who view motherhood as a cultural trap (Jones & Mitchell, as cited in Allison, 1979). Women have worked for over 100 years for the right to limit fertility, thus fighting to *have* children has been a less vocal, lower priority issue that affects far fewer women. For some feminists, "the wish for children reflects oppressive social conditioning" as well as a depletion of limited resources (Doyal, 1987, p. 186). Bardwick (1971) claimed that motherhood is always an ambivalent part of women's lives; infertility can heighten that sense of confusion.

Historically, male infertility was assumed to indicate subpar virility; to counter such potential social judgments, many women falsely claim that the infertility problem is their own in order to protect their husband's image. An Israeli woman said,

> I am not ready to admit my husband has a low sperm count. It is too hard on him, he has suffered enough humiliation in the course of the treatment. I usually say that my tubes are closed–it's no one's fault, and it stops further questions. Many people anyway think infertility is a woman's problem. (Remennick, 2000, p. 832)

Men are, in fact, no less distressed by a medical diagnosis of infertility than women are (Edelmann & Connolly, 2000), but they express it far differently. They are more likely to see it as an affront to their sense of virility or as an inability to continue the family name; it is less likely to be about the absence of the father role, although that is sometimes also present. More data need to be obtained; presently much of it is "derived from interviews," which overrepresent women because of their "tendency to express their feelings more readily to a stranger" (Edelmann & Connolly, 2000, pp. 372-3). According to Griel (1991), "husbands are less likely . . . to [see] themselves as having spoiled identity" but rather "as having bodily failure" (p. 6).

PRIVACY ISSUES

For many reasons, including its inextricable ties with sexuality and sense of shame or stigma, many women and couples choose to maintain a façade to their friends and families by implying that they are childless by choice. Infertility is a hidden condition, generally; the only "proof" is lack of children, and there are many voluntary reasons why couples defer or omit parenting. The change from private to public occurs only with "selective disclosure" or "information management" (Goffman, 1963, p. 57), that is, deciding which parts of the story to tell and with what "spin."

However, the very act of seeking out medical treatment may interfere with the individual's ability to keep this information truly private (Kirkman, 2001). This includes the very real need to miss work or other obligations because of the frequency and exquisite timing of infertility evaluation appointments and the inability to sustain alternative excuses for these absences (Griel, 1991; Kirkman, 2001).

In working with this population, the therapist must help couples determine what are appropriate boundaries. Therapists can help not only in the definition but also in the enforcement of boundaries. This is a key feature in negotiating with all the couple's friends and family members, especially those who are the parents of young children. Boundaries will help infertile patients assess how to participate, or abstain, from all the rituals and ceremonies attendant to the childhood milestones. Boundaries will also help them to answer, or deflect, the questions and unsolicited advice about fertility plans and procedures that may seem intrusive and unwelcome.

COPING WITH OTHERS' RITES OF PASSAGE

Whether one is public or private about the reasons for one's childlessness, other people have children and all the attendant rituals associated with them (baby showers, christenings, bris, baby namings, juvenile birthdays), which infertile people are often expected to attend. Infertile people may be central to the event (e.g., as godparents) or peripheral (e.g., as co-workers), and they may need some help deciding which events are required and which, because of too much pain, may be omitted. Often, women and couples use "strategic avoidance" (Kohler Riessman, 2000, p. 123). They select events where there will be other childless people or where there are less likely to be people who will question them about their future fertility and family plans.

When a couple is childless, there are certain lifestyle advantages because of fewer fixed expenses and less constrained scheduling. To the outside world, it may seem that the couple has chosen extravagant vacations and frequent restaurant dinners instead of diapers, playgroups, and babysitter dilemmas. To the couple, the compensation of such alternatives is often inadequate for the pain and loss they feel as outsiders to the parenting cohort.

LOSS OF ROLE

Infertility may be a form of stigma or "spoiled identity" (Goffman, 1963) for infertile women because motherhood is so often a central role, whether within the larger unit of a pronatalist society, a smaller social unit (family, friends, or community), or within her own self-definition. The role identity is correlated with gender stereotypes, which result from observations of people behaving "appropriately" within their social roles (Prentice & Miller, 2002). People develop both "personal identities" that define individuals in relation to other individuals and "social identities that derive from memberships in emotionally significant social groups" (Prentice & Miller, p. 353).

In some women's reference groups, to omit the role of mother may be perceived not only as deviant but as a pointless existence. In India, for example, "sexual reproduction allows for social reproduction" among families of wealth and property (Kohler Riessman, 2000, p. 112); motherhood is a matter not only of "psychological or sentimental discourses" but also of "critical cultural discourses" (p. 112). In the United States, for women who have limited educational or career opportunities or interests, the role of mother can offer an enhanced status in relation to the occupational milieu in which they are likely to find themselves. Not to be a mother, then, may relegate these women to unwanted continued employment, as well as diminished status within the extended family network.

One of the tasks for therapists is to help each women decide what the meaning of motherhood is for her, apart from her sense of what it should be. Motherhood is a complex role, and there are many ways to be successful in it . . . or without it.

TRANSITION FROM HEALTHY/NORMAL
TO SICK/ABNORMAL

Most infertile women and men have presumed themselves healthy for most of their lives and assumed that their reproductive potential was normal, until they tried to conceive and could not. It is often a long process for people to discontinue "trying" each month and assuming it will "just happen" to acknowledging that there is a problem that will require medical intervention. It is a sea change to make the transition from healthy person to person who needs extensive, intensive, protracted, and expensive medical evaluation and treatment. It is very hard to go from loving spouse and incipient parent to infertility patient.

If the treatment includes fertility drugs, women have to cope with the many unpleasant physiological side effects that often exacerbate psychological fragility, and a woman's functioning is frequently compromised, which adds more stress to what is likely an already strained relationship with her partner. Furthermore, although most infertile women will choose to utilize these drugs, it is unclear what the long-term effects of such high dosage hormones will be on future health.

Many of the drugs work by overstimulating the ovaries, which often results in multiple fetuses. Drugs can cause a high-risk pregnancy, a greater likelihood of fetal death, and birth defects in the resulting children, thus the couple faces great emotional stress. Therapists have to help patients cope with the emotional roller coaster of multiple fetuses, which are often "discovered" on sonograms at different times in the early weeks, decisions about what is referred to as fetal reduction, and the potential spontaneous fetal loss. Even if all goes well, the couple must cope with the very real exigencies of multiple births, including protracted bed rest or hospitalization during the pregnancy.

It is less likely today, but up until the 1970s women with unexplained infertility were given a diagnosis of psychogenic infertility, which effectively blamed a woman for her own infertility. Physicians, who lacked sufficient biological knowledge, assigned the etiology to a woman's mental health status; thus they erred by seeing her distress as causative rather than as a result of the infertility (Menning, 1977; Spector, 1985; Unruh & McGrath, 1985).

The therapist's role here is very similar to the role with victims of sexual abuse who were blamed for their circumstances. It is imperative that women see that depression and anxiety most often result *from* infertility; there is no scientific evidence to demonstrate that they are etiologically significant.

THE RELATIONSHIP WITH THE MEDICAL SYSTEM AND QUALITY OF CARE

The therapist has an important role to validate the emotional, social, and physical difficulties of the infertility treatment. Thus, therapists should have a working knowledge of the medical style and approach of infertility specialists in general and, where possible, of the specific personalities within her community. Patients should feel justified in rejecting practitioners who are arrogant, authoritarian, and uncaring, and in setting and enforcing their own standards for treatment options.

> He is the only doctor I know who can do a pelvic with one foot out the door. And the fact that he is prestigious and important makes me feel I cannot call him or demand anything more than what he gives me. (Menning, 1977, p. 156)

> It's like going through a battery team. You get about 30 seconds with the doctor who doesn't really sit down. . . . (Pfeffer & Woollett, as cited in Doyal, 1987, p. 183)

> On the second visit, the psychiatrist said to me, "I appreciate you've been through a lot but I just don't quite understand why you're *so* upset because your miscarriage happened several years ago." (Kirkman, 2001, p. 531)

Patients also need to understand that medical terminology can sound harsh to the ears of the uninitiated, but that it is physicians' jargon and not meant to be offensive. Although the physicians refer to the entity as a conceptus or an embryo or a fetus, the woman or couple may see it as a baby or a potential baby. When a spontaneous abortion occurs, a layperson refers to it as a miscarriage, or a loss of baby; the medical staff considers it the "product of conception" or "pregnancy wastage."

For most couples, it will be an asset to attend as many medical appointments together as possible, not only to provide emotional support, but to ask all the necessary questions and to have more than one person who can remember the answers. It is helpful for patients to attend appointments with all questions and concerns in writing, so that they remember to address all of them with the physician, and to write down the answers; the anxiety of the situation often interferes with accurate information processing and retrieval. Taking notes will also aid in compliance with whatever regimen is suggested by the physician.

For the couple, working together with a psychotherapist is an adjunct to the medical process. It provides an opportunity to articulate the difficulties that arise, both within the couple and with the medical system and remedies. This enables the couple to resolve the problems, work together (which strengthens the couple's relationship), and have the energy and focus to address the remaining obstacles. For example, if a couple is not adhering to the schedule for taking the basal body temperature or having sexual intercourse timed to maximize conception, the therapist can help them to examine and resolve the underlying ambivalence or unconscious conflict that may be at the root of the problem.

The patient's personality and affect also influences the quality of medical care and his or her perception of that care. It begins with the physician's attitudes toward the woman, demographically and emotionally–is this an "appropriate" woman or couple to reproduce? Sexual, racial, and class biases affect the physicians' views about access to treatment, whether the physician is aware of them or not. Physicians do not like to fail; it may be psychologically more comfortable for them to shift the blame onto the patient (consciously or unconsciously) and to decide (directly or indirectly) to discontinue treatment or to discourage the person from continuing treatment. That way, the treatment is an incomplete trial rather than an unsuccessful one.

> The American Medical Association's ethical guidelines say that, except in emergencies, a physician may choose whom to treat. This permits the physician to apply his/her skills where he/she wants to but also protects the patient. Good medical care requires the doctor and the patient to establish an intimate ongoing relationship of trust. This is not possible if the physician is seething with resentment. (Cohen, 2001, p. 18)

A passive, needy woman may either irritate the doctor and the medical staff or she may be perceived as an appropriately feminine, "motherly" woman. An assertive, goal-oriented woman, especially one who gathers information on her own, may be seen as a partner in the infertility treatment or as an adversary in a power struggle. It can be a question of "Who owns the medical information?" Medical sociologist Eliot Friedson (1970) wrote that physicians all too often *give* information *to* patients but seldom *ask* for information *from* patients. Whereas women may feel and act as if they have the right to control their own bodies and participate in their own health care (Unruh & McGrath, 1985), some doctors may "resist mutual participation" (p. 374). For these reasons, as well as the fee-for-service model, patients should be encouraged to be active and educated consumers, to search out not only medically successful practices, but also compassionate and respectful care. Although selecting one's own physician is still the ideal treatment model, managed care and cost containment has precluded that for many infertility patients.

More than 25 years ago, Menning (1977) advocated a team approach of various professional disciplines to manage both the physical and emotional issues of infertile couples. This is still an optimum care model, although economics rarely makes it feasible. As one alternative to a team of specialists and a way of gathering resources for information and support, therapists can recommend various Websites to their patients (see Appendix).

CLOSURE

The therapist has the responsibility to assist in the mourning process, not only the process of mourning for the child that never was and never will be, but for the parents that may never be. In that sense, "it is the death of a dream. There are no solid things to remember (about the pregnancy or the child) because he [sic] never existed" (Menning, 1977, p. 130).

Childless and childfree both signify no children, but their emotional tones are far different from one another. Therapists can help patients to decide which definition to apply to themselves, as well as deciding whether to "speed up" or "shut down" the infertility treatment juggernaut. Couples often need a lot of therapeutic support to decide which avenue to pursue: childless lifestyle or adoption.

Two of the ways to resolve infertility are to become pregnant or to adopt a baby. The choice may depend on to what extent the people are child-oriented or pregnancy-oriented (Menning, 1977, pp. 100-102). Pregnancy represents genetic continuity, proof of virility, narcissism, and the wish to experience pregnancy-related bodily changes (including breastfeeding). It is also a way to "balance out the previous pregnancy failures and losses" (Menning, 1977, p. 100). For many infertile and fertile couples, it is an attempt to enhance their relationship.

Having waited so long to be parents, and often relegated to one child, people often believe they have to become "superparents" who not only provide everything for the child but who cannot verbalize any of the normal complaints that parents have about childrearing.

> I waited so long to be a mother and my twins mean everything to me. How can I say I am too tired to get up to feed them, or that their incessant crying is driving me crazy? I am so lucky to have them. I feel ungrateful if I complain. (Menning, 1977, p. 100)

If the couple has used any of the Assisted Reproductive Technologies (ART), there may be other issues for the couple to address. If a sperm or egg donor has been used, and only one parent will be biologically related to the child, issues of unbalanced genetic connection must be balanced against the desire to achieve a pregnancy and have a child from infancy. They can look "normal" to others even if the couple does not feel truly normal in the way the pregnancy was created. This covert information raises, again, the couple's privacy boundaries: Do they tell others? Do they tell their child? And will it affect the nonrelated person's relationship with the child? Will the child be viewed as belonging more to one person than the other?

Couples may, of course, choose to adopt, with all the difficulties inherent in a system that has so few available healthy infants for those who want them. There are many adoption options: public or private, domestic or foreign, older child, special needs child. Each has its benefits and deficits, but all generally take a long time and exact large financial and emotional costs. However, if the couple obtains an "appropriate" child, it is all worth it.

For many infertile people, grieving the loss of the potential baby (whether not conceived or carried to term) is not one loss nor does it have a predictable or easily definable time schedule. It is ongoing and recurring. Patients have to make the decision(s) about continuing or discontinuing the medical process; they may stop and start again more than once as they grapple with the grueling process of trying to have a baby (Borg & Lasker, 1981; Lasker & Borg, 1987). Fertility is not lost but reduced and elusive; the hope for the anticipated and much wanted child(ren) remains, but, for some, always out of reach (Unruh & McGrath, 1985).

Infertility is a constant struggle between hope and failure. The appearance (again and again) of menstrual blood, the blood of a potential or actual spontaneous abortion, medical evidence that one is anovulatory, the arrival of menopause, erectile dysfunction, the evidence that one is azoospermatic, or repeated treatment failures (e.g., in vitro fertilization), as well as the abandonment by the medical authority ("We think you are too old to keep trying") all suggest to patients that they should end the quest for the biological baby. Having invested a lifetime of assuming and hoping, and years of a single-minded focus of trying to achieve a successful pregnancy, it is very hard to terminate the process and have "nothing to show for all that effort" (Remennick, 2000, p. 836). Yet, it may be the correct choice for them, and they may need substantial help from their therapist to close this protracted chapter in their lives and assess how to write the rest of their story.

For some, it may mean developing and maintaining close relationships with the children of friends or relatives or becoming foster parents. Some people may choose to have children in their lives by volunteer activities or by changing careers. For others, it may mean moving into a less child-oriented world so that they have little contact with children. The therapist's task is to help each person take the time to mourn, recover, and select the strategy that is the most appropriate, based on the person's history, developmental stage, present level of functioning, and future goals. Infertile patients come to the office with a myriad of problems, some clearly related to the specifics of their current medical problem and loss of social role, some more subtle and complicated. Therapy may continue through the diagnosis and acceptance of the infertility through closure, as well as beyond.

REFERENCES

Allison, J. R. (1979). Roles and role conflict of women in infertile couples. *Psychology of Women Quarterly*, *4*, 97-113.

Bardwick, J. M. (1971). *The psychology of women: A study of bio-cultural conflicts.* New York: Harper & Row.

Bernard, J. (1974). *The future of motherhood.* New York: Penguin Books.

Borg, S., & Lasker, J. (1981). *When pregnancy fails: Families coping with miscarriage, still birth, and infant death.* Boston: Beacon Press.

Cohen, R. (2001, December 23). The ethicist. *New York Times Magazine*, p. 18.

Dorland's Medical Dictionary (2000). Philadelphia: Saunders.

Doyal, L. (1987). Infertility–a life sentence? Women and the National Health Service. In M. Stanorth (Ed.), *Reproductive technologies: Gender, motherhood, and medicine* (pp. 175-190). Minneapolis: University of Minnesota Press.

Edelmann, R. J., & Connolly, K. J. (2000). Gender differences in response to infertility and infertility investigations: Real or illusory. *British Journal of Health Psychology*, *5*, 365-375.

Freeman, E. W., Boxer, A. S., Rickels, K., Tureck, R., & Mastrioanni, L. (1985). Psychological evaluation and support in a program of in vitro fertilization and embryo transfer. *Fertility and Sterility*, *43*, 48-53.

Friedson, E. (1970). *Profession of medicine: A study in the sociology of applied knowledge.* New York: Dodd, Mead.

Goffman, E. (1963). *Stigma: Notes on the management of spoiled identity.* Englewood Cliffs, NJ: Prentice-Hall.

Griel, A. L. (1991). *Not yet pregnant: Infertile couples in contemporary America.* New Brunswick, NJ: Rutgers University Press.

Kirkman, M. (2001). Thinking of something to say: Public and private narratives of infertility. *Health Care for Women International, 22,* 523-535.

Kohler Riessman, C. (2000). Stigma and everyday resistance practices: Childless women in South India. *Gender & Society, 14,* 111-135.

Lasker, J. M., & Borg, S. (1987). *In search of parenthood: Coping with infertility and high-tech conception.* Boston: Beacon Press.

Marsh, M. (1997). Motherhood denied: Women and infertility in historical perspective. In R. D. Apple & J. Golden (Eds.), *Mothers and motherhood* (pp. 216-241). Columbus, OH: Ohio State University.

Menning, B. E. (1977). *Infertility: A guide for the childless couple.* Englewood Cliffs, NJ: Prentice-Hall.

Mosher, W. D. & Pratt, W. F. (1982). *Reproductive impairments among married couples: United States.* (Vital and Health Statistics, Public Health Service, 23, 1-51). Washington, DC: U.S. Government Printing Office.

Polit, D. F. (1978). Stereotypes relating to family-size status. *Journal of Marriage and the Family, 40,* 105-114.

Poston, D. L. Jr., & Kramer, K. B.(1980). Characteristics of voluntarily and involuntarily childless wives. Unpublished paper, Population Research Center, University of Texas, Austin, TX.

Prentice, D. A., & Miller, D. T. (2002). The emergence of homegrown stereotypes. *American Psychologist, 57,* 323-359.

Remennick, L. (2000). Childless in the land of imperative motherhood: Stigma and coping among infertile Israeli women. *Sex Roles, 43,* 821-841.

Rosenberg, C. E., & Smith-Rosenberg, C. (1976). The female animal: Medical and biological views of women. In C. E. Rosenberg (Ed.), *No other gods: On science and American social thought* (pp. 54-70). Baltimore: Johns Hopkins University Press.

Russo, N. F. (1979). Overview: Sex roles, fertility, and the motherhood mandate. *Psychology of Women Quarterly, 4,* 7-15.

Scharf, C. N., & Weinshel, M. (2001). Infertility and late-life pregnancies. In P. Papp (Ed.), *Couples on the fault line* (pp. 104-129). New York: Guilford Press.

Spector, A. R. (1985). *Effects of fertility status on women's self-concept and life choices.* Unpublished doctoral dissertation, University of Pennsylvania.

Unruh, A. M., & McGrath, P. J. (1985). The psychology of female infertility: Toward a new perspective. *Health Care for Women International, 6,* 369-381.

Whelpton, P. K., Campbell, A. A., & Patterson, J. E. (1966). *Fertility and family planning in the United States.* Princeton, NJ: Princeton University Press.

Williams, L. S., & Power, P. W. (1977). The emotional impact of infertility in single women: Some implications for counseling. *Journal of the American Medical Women's Association, 51/53,* 327-333.

APPENDIX

Websites

American College of Obstetricians and Gynecology
http://www.acog.org/

Pregnancy Today: ACOG Guidelines
http://pregnancytoday.com/references/articles/

American Society for Reproductive Medicine
http://www.asrm.org

Assisted Reproductive Technology (ART)
http://www.resolvemn.org/art.htm

Assisted Reproductive Technologies-HSPH
http://www.hsph.harvard.edu/Organizations/healthnet

ASRM: Ethical Considerations of ART
http://www.asrm.org/Media/Ethics/ethicsmain.html

Infertility: Infertility Info at iVillage.com
http://www.ivillage.com/topics/family/infertility/

RESOLVE: The National Infertility Association
http://www.resolve.org/

Society for Reproductive Endocrinology and Infertility
http://www.socrei.org/SREImap.html

Reproductive Endocrinology
http://members.aol.com/fertilmd/

The Aftermath of Pregnancy Loss: A Feminist Critique of the Literature and Implications for Treatment

Lisa Cosgrove

SUMMARY. Although 15%-20% of pregnancies end in miscarriage (Borg & Lasker, 1989; Swanson, 1999), many health care professionals do not recognize miscarriage as a psychologically taxing event, and thus women are not routinely provided with follow-up care (Lee, Slade, & Lygo, 1996; Reinharz, 1988). The purpose of this article is to explore some of the issues that arise for women who experience pregnancy loss and to offer some suggestions for therapists working with women and their families. The psychological literature on perinatal loss is reviewed from a critical feminist perspective. I argue that therapists must privilege the personal meanings of a woman's stillbirth or miscarriage experience, while simultaneously appreciating the sociopolitical context in which the loss is embedded. *[Article copies available for a fee from The Haworth Document Delivery Service: 1-800-HAWORTH. E-mail address: <docdelivery@haworthpress.com>*

Lisa Cosgrove, PhD, is Assistant Professor, Department of Counseling and School Psychology, University of Massachusetts at Boston. She has published articles and book chapters on critical psychology, research methods, community psychology, feminist therapy, and the implications of postmodernism for feminist research and practice. She also has a private practice in Natick, Massachusetts.

Address correspondence to: Lisa Cosgrove, Department of Counseling and School Psychology, University of Massachusetts at Boston, 100 Morrissey Blvd., Boston, MA 01215-3393 (E-mail: lisa.cosgrove@umb.edu).

[Haworth co-indexing entry note]: "The Aftermath of Pregnancy Loss: A Feminist Critique of the Literature and Implications for Treatment." Cosgrove, Lisa. Co-published simultaneously in *Women & Therapy* (The Haworth Press, Inc.) Vol. 27, No. 3/4, 2004, pp. 107-122; and: *From Menarche to Menopause: The Female Body in Feminist Therapy* (ed: Joan C. Chrisler) The Haworth Press, Inc., 2004, pp. 107-122. Single or multiple copies of this article are available for a fee from The Haworth Document Delivery Service [1-800-HAWORTH, 9:00 a.m. - 5:00 p.m. (EST). E-mail address: docdelivery@haworthpress.com].

10.1300/J015v27n03_08

KEYWORDS. Miscarriage, feminist therapy, pregnancy loss

Although women generally do not expect to miscarry and are shocked when they do (Reinharz, 1988), miscarriage is actually a more common event than most people realize. Estimates[1] are usually in the 15%-20% range for clinically recognized pregnancies (Borg & Lasker, 1989; Swanson, 1999) and 31% for total pregnancy loss after implantation, i.e., including pregnancies that are not clinically recognized (Wilcox et al., 1988). In women over age 40 the risk for miscarriage dramatically increases to over 60% (Chung & Yeko, 1996). Stillbirths are far less common than miscarriages. They account for approximately 1% of all births; however, this translates into at least 33,000 stillbirths each year (DeFrain, Martens, Stork, & Stork, 1990). As these statistics demonstrate (and especially in light of the fact that more women are choosing to have children later in life), it is very likely that therapists will have clients who have experienced a pregnancy loss. Indeed, as Glazer (1997) noted, "[w]ith increasingly sophisticated technological options for fostering conception, miscarriage has become a more frequent event for scores of couples who previously might not even have known they were pregnant" (p. 230). In this article I provide a brief review of the literature on the emotional aftermath of miscarriage and stillbirth, identify some problematic assumptions and conclusions of existing research, and offer some specific suggestions for therapists working with women who have experienced perinatal loss. Particular attention will be paid to the ways in which the medicalization of pregnancy, and the female body more generally, impacts on the aftermath of pregnancy loss.

DEFINITION OF TERMS

The medicalized female body, constituted as an object of interest for the medical gaze, is removed from the social and ideological contexts in which it is lived and interpreted.

–Zita (1988)

The vocabulary that health care professionals use to describe reproductive functioning and pregnancy loss reveals assumptions not only about the female body and reproductivity but also about how women who experience pregnancy loss should be "managed." Indeed, an all too frequent complaint voiced by women is that the language used to describe pregnancy loss either fails to capture, or runs in stark contrast to, their miscarriage or stillbirth experiences. Therefore, it is imperative for therapists to be familiar with the terms typically used by health care professionals. But familiarity and even critique are not enough; we must also deconstruct the biomedical discourse to which women are subjected (i.e., examine the hidden assumptions of this discourse). First, I will briefly define some of the terms that are commonly used to describe pregnancy loss by medical professionals, then I will discuss the ways in which this discourse medicalizes the female body and undermines an appreciation for women's lived experience of pregnancy loss.

Chemical pregnancy: A pregnancy that is announced by sensitive assays for hCG in the blood or by ultrasound when a woman uses assisted reproduction and is closely monitored (Glazer, 1997).

Spontaneous abortion: The unintended ending of a pregnancy before the fetus can survive outside the womb. This event is more commonly referred to as a miscarriage by nonmedical personnel.

Missed abortion: Occurs when a fetus dies in utero but there are no symptoms such as cramping, spotting, or bleeding.

Late abortion or premature fetus: A pregnancy in which the fetus dies after the 26th week. The specific term used depends on the weight of the fetus (Shapiro, 1993).

Habitual aborters: Women who have multiple miscarriages.

Stillbirth: The death of a fetus between the 20th week of pregnancy and birth.

It has been documented that "few hospitals train [health care providers] or even have a well-thought out policy on the management of miscarriage" (Moulder, 1994, p. 65), which perhaps is not surprising when one considers how the medical model conceptualizes pregnancy loss. That is, as is evident from the terms noted above, the medical model sees miscarriage as a minor emergency that can be treated in a routine way; the *physical* management of miscarriage has an accepted and standardized protocol. Moreover, as Glazer (1997) pointed out, the label "chemical pregnancy" has prompted some health care personnel to differentiate between two categories of miscarriages: physical and technological. The former is distinguished from the latter by "bleeding, cramping, or the sudden loss of pregnancy symptoms" (p. 238). From a biomedical standpoint, a "technological" miscarriage is a lesser "routine emergency" than a physical one, and, unfortunately, it is usually treated as a lesser loss. However, as Glazer noted:

> Women who experience a "technological" miscarriage (especially if it is referred to as "just a chemical pregnancy") are confused by what has happened. . . . [From] an emotional standpoint a "technological" miscarriage can be more difficult and challenging than a physical miscarriage. Although the latter is painful emotionally as well as physically, the women who experience a miscarriage in which there are observable

physical changes have some sense that a natural process, however upsetting, is occurring. Their loss is real, concrete, and identifiable. (p. 238)

Within the framework of the medical model, there is a tendency to conflate increased physical complexity with increased emotional complexity, which gives rise to the belief that grieving will be more intense the longer the duration of the pregnancy. The assumption that the later in gestation that the loss occurs, the more intense the grief reaction will be (see, for example, Beil, 1992) is buoyed by the medical discourse and terms noted above, and sustained by the erroneous belief that the mother becomes increasingly attached to the child as the fetus grows physically bigger. However, the aftermath of pregnancy loss is a complex experience, and the level of distress should not be conflated with gestation stage (Moulder, 1994). It is the *meaning* that women give to their pregnancies and their individual histories that are crucial in shaping their experience of perinatal loss: "Women miscarrying at the same gestational stage can react very differently depending on their own definition of the experience . . . [on the other hand] a woman in her twenties, the mother of two children who miscarries at 22 weeks may react with similar intensity to a woman in her late thirties with fertility problems who finally conceives only to miscarry at 8 weeks" (Moulder, 1994, p. 66). Indeed, there is very little substantive evidence to suggest any impact of duration of gestation for women who experience miscarriage (Slade, 1994; Thapar & Thapar, 1992). In fact, some researchers (e.g., Peppers & Knapp, 1980) found that women who had miscarried scored as high on an assessment of emotional distress as did women who had delivered a stillborn child. In addition, Leppert and Pahlka (1984) reported that the grief reaction following a miscarriage was as intense as that found in women who had experienced a stillbirth or neonatal death.

The conflation of distress with gestational stage not only lacks empirical verification, but it also flies in the face of technology; an intense early bonding experience is made possible by the visual image (and ultrasound picture) of one's fetus. Thus, the increased role of technology may complicate and exacerbate the "disenfranchised grief" (Doka, 1989) of pregnancy loss. As Petchesky (1987) noted in her feminist analysis of fetal images, we live in a visually oriented culture, and a woman may experience an increased attachment to her child at a very early stage of pregnancy because of fetal imaging techniques. Also, it has been suggested that fetal imaging "may enhance the desired participation in . . . the pregnancy by partners (who may be men or women)" (Harding, 1998, p. 32). However, in the event of pregnancy loss, it is unclear whether the bonding made possible via technology helps or hinders a woman and/or her partner in coming to terms with the loss (Cecil, 1994).

Not only have scientific and medical discourses failed to appreciate women's lived experiences, but they have also sustained the mind/body dualism and "contributed to the fragmentation of the unity of the person by treating the body as a machine to be fixed by the physician-as-technician" (Martin,

1987, as cited in Harding, 1998, p. 95). Medical terms such as chemical pregnancy, premature fetus, and spontaneous abortion do not simply undermine an appreciation for women's experience; the vocabularies used to describe the experience (e.g., by medical personnel) *create* certain realities and experiences and marginalize others (Burr, 1995; Cosgrove, 2000; Gergen, 1994). Biomedical discourse is a constituting activity that involves the production of power and (what counts as) knowledge, and as such it (re)produces a female subject and medicalized body in constant need of surveillance and regulation (Cosgrove & Riddle, 2003; Fausto-Sterling, 2000; Harding, 1998; Martin, 1987; Smart, 1992; Ussher, 1996; Zita, 1988). Thus, health care professionals' vocabularies are not simply neutral acts of description that engender an "objective"–but helpful–response to women who have experienced a pregnancy loss. In fact, "the medical model focuses on the event as a minor mishap which can be treated (ERPC, Evacuation of the Retained Products of Conception) and cured (try again in 1-3 months). There is no mention of a pregnancy, a baby, and any element of loss is ignored" (Moulder, 1994, p. 65; see also Reinharz, 1988). Indeed, a "spontaneous abortion" is a clinical entity, something to be effectively "treated" by dispassionate attention to the vaginal exam (ERPC) and by "making the womb an object of power/knowledge, plac[ing] the womb under surveillance, monitor[ing] and control[ing] it" (Harding, 1998, p. 32). A "miscarriage," on the other hand, is an intra- and interpersonal experience to which one should respond with empathy and care.

REVIEW OF THE LITERATURE: IDENTIFYING CONCEPTUAL AND METHODOLOGICAL PROBLEMS

Prior to the 1990s very few empirical studies were conducted on the psychological impact of pregnancy loss (Beil, 1992). The few published studies prior to this time tended to be psychoanalytic in orientation, relied on very limited case studies, and focused on the psychogenic origins of miscarriage. The authors of these articles made egregiously sexist assumptions and engaged in blatant victim-blame. For example, "habitual aborters" (the medical term used to describe women who had recurrent miscarriages) were described as having "infantile personalities with confused sex identity" (Weil & Tupper, 1960), "autonomic instability" (Dunbar, 1954), or ambivalence about (or outright rejection of) motherhood (Hertz, 1973). One physician even went so far as to conclude that "habitual aborters" tend to be "frigid . . . and develop an abortion habit just as others develop an accident habit, [but] this habit may be interrupted by well-directed psychosomatic treatment" (Squier & Dunbar, 1946, p. 174). Weil and Tupper (1960) claimed that the "aborters" in their study, "despite their air of aloofness tolerate[d] any kind of stress badly. Pregnancy . . . brought about fantasies of feminine attainment, but at the same time threatened them with an emotional attachment to a baby toward which they would also have liked to feel "the hell with it" (p. 450). Similarly, Hertz (1973) concluded that "these women" demonstrate "faulty anticipations and acting out behavior [because of their ambivalence about motherhood]. It seems that as the world did not want them on their terms, they rejected the world–including pregnancy" (p. 243).

Unfortunately however, the blatant sexism evidenced in the psychological literature on pregnancy loss from the 1940s through the 1970s has not been replaced with a fully feminist understanding of the female body, reproductive functioning, and ideologies of motherhood. The majority of the empirically based literature focuses almost exclusively on identifying variables that can best predict the level and type of distress following pregnancy loss and on "managing" miscarriage. The focus on control and prediction is certainly not surprising; indeed, it is the legacy of the positivist epistemology that grounds the discipline of psychology. However, the positivist framework is deeply problematic for a number of reasons. First, insofar as such a framework privileges measurement over description, it distorts experience for "emotional pain defies objective measurement" (DeFrain, 1991, p. 230). Despite the fact that there have been a number of studies over the last 10 years that have examined the psychological sequelae of pregnancy loss, those studies have not captured the depth and complexity of this experience.

Second, the instruments used to assess affective responses to pregnancy loss tend to reify grief and pathologize other emotional responses such as depression and anxiety. The reification of emotional responses leads researchers to look for intra-individual explanations for these emotions. For example, a number of researchers found, not surprisingly, that depression and anxiety are common responses following a perinatal loss. This finding has led researchers to design studies to find out what intra-individual factors (e.g., "pre-loss neurotic personality," Janssen, Cuisiner, de Graauw, & Hoogduin, 1997) best predict levels of depression.

Not only does the tendency to look for intra-individual factors to explain experience and distress foster victim blame (Fine, 1992), but such an approach also fails to appreciate the ways in which women *are* held responsible for the "success" of their pregnancies. Gardner (1995) summed this up well when she described the cultural representations and lived experience of pregnancy in terms of a "rhetoric of fetal endangerment." Also, as Armstrong (2000) pointed out, the role of formal and informal "education" in the experience of pregnancy has increased dramatically in recent years. She wrote that "the key elements of this frame are notions of control and responsibility for [pregnancy] outcome . . . [there has been a] public health shift from an emphasis on societal responsibility for ensuring healthy babies to individual responsibility (and especially culpability for unwanted outcomes) making women's behavior during pregnancy the target of intense personal and political scrutiny" (p. 587).

In light of the way in which the medical management of pregnancy has become normalized (Armstrong, 2000; Gardner, 1995; Markens, Browner, & Press, 1997) it is not surprising that women who experience perinatal loss scrutinize their behavior during pregnancy and engage in self-recrimination and guilt over things such as sexual activity, what they should (or should not) have eaten, or the amount and intensity of exercise in which they should (or should not) have engaged. Unfortunately, however, researchers have not paid adequate attention to the ways in which dominant discourses, rhetoric, and practices sustain feelings of guilt, anxiety, or self-recrimination.[2] Instead, researchers try to identify personality characteristics or demographic variables that predict such feelings (see, for example, Friedman & Gath, 1989; Murray & Callan, 1988; Prettyman, Cordle, & Cook, 1993; Slade, 1994). Thus, it is all too common for investigators to ground their research in questions such as: "Is the personality trait 'neuroticism,' predictive of pathological grief disturbances following perinatal loss?" (see, for example, Janssen et al., 1997). Insofar as researchers try to account for anxiety and guilt via intra-individual factors, the subtle but powerful ways in which anxiety and feelings of self-recrimination *are produced* by dominant discourses and practices becomes obscured. Moreover, the normalization of the medical management of pregnancy "indicates acceptance of the growing emphasis on the exclusive or nearly exclusive role of maternal responsibility for fetal outcome. . . . [This emphasis] contrasts sharply with the reality of poverty and environmental hazards that feminist activists and other health advocates argue are more significant in explaining pregnancy outcomes" (Markens et al., 1997, p. 369).

It should also be noted that the positivist focus on controlling and predicting variables also renders invisible the myriad of ways in which coping and emotional resilience can be manifest. For example, many researchers (e.g., Beil, 1992) accept concepts such as "avoidant coping" as unproblematic. However, what may be instrumentalized as "avoidant" or "dysfunctional" coping by the psychological researcher may be *experienced* as a strategic and helpful way of coping by the participant (especially if the participant is disenfranchised and marginalized by race, class, or sexual orientation). As Fine (1992) argued, "psychologists have prescribed ways to cope as if a consensus about their utility had been established . . . and as if these strategies were uninfluenced by our position in social and economic hierarchies" (p. 70).

An additional limitation of the literature on the aftermath of pregnancy loss is the way in which assumptions about compulsory heterosexuality inform research agendas and conclusions. Despite awareness that technological advances have allowed many women to get pregnant who previously would not have been able to, the voices of single or lesbian mothers and nontraditional couples are nowhere to be found in the research literature. By failing to consider the ways in which implicit assumptions about compulsory heterosexuality determine the focus of their work, researchers have actively silenced the experiences of many women and their partners. This is an obvious gap in the literature, and one that must be addressed so that "women's responses" to pregnancy loss are not conflated with "married heterosexual women's responses to pregnancy loss."

CONTRIBUTIONS OF RECENT RESEARCH

Over 14 years ago, Reinharz (1988) wrote that the invisibility of miscarriage can be seen clearly by the use of the word "fetus." Researchers "focus on fetuses rather than on women; they examine the etiology of the demise of the fetuses rather than the history of the woman's relation with her dead baby" (1988, p. 85). Although it is still true that studies on the epidemiology and etiology of miscarriage far outnumber those on the aftermath experience, some important contributions have been made. For example, the literature suggests that demographic variables such as maternal age and social or occupational class are unhelpful predictors of type or level of distress[3] (Slade, 1994; Lee, Slade, & Lygo, 1996). Also, there is little support for the assumption that miscarriage leads to fewer negative emotional consequences if a woman already has children (Slade, 1994).

There is also consensus about the frequency of depressive symptoms following a pregnancy loss. In a very thorough review of the quantitative evidence concerning the psychological impact of miscarriage, Slade (1994) reported that between 20-50% of women experience "significant depressive symptoms within the first month after a miscarriage" (p. 7). Anxiety has been less well-studied, which led Slade to conclude that the frequency of anxiety is not known and "the temporal patterning for anxiety symptoms may be more complex [than for depressive symptoms]" (p. 7). The role of anger as an outcome of pregnancy loss is now beginning to receive attention, in part due to the widespread recognition that anger is experienced by many, if not most, people who experience significant loss. Swanson's (1999) preliminary work suggests that there is a clear "link between making meaning of just what was lost and the experience of anger" (p. 196). It is critical for women to recognize the legitimacy and importance of anger in the healing process; however, it appears that unresolved anger exacerbates feelings of hopelessness and constrains one's future.

The empirical literature has also contributed to an increased awareness of the significance of health care providers' attitudes toward pregnancy loss and, concomitantly, of how these attitudes impact on the care provided to women. How medical personnel and obstetric teams respond following miscarriage and stillbirth often has a profound effect on the aftermath of pregnancy loss (Condon, 1986; Prettyman & Cordle, 1992; Rajan & Oakley, 1993; Swanson, 1999; Thapar & Thapar, 1992). For example, women report feeling disappointed, isolated, and/or silenced by the emotional unavailability of medical personnel (Cecil, 1994; Kirkley-Best & Kellner, 1982; Rajan & Oakley,

1993). Although more research is needed regarding what women want most from their health care team, the existing literature suggests that empathic responses by health care personnel facilitate the grieving process. Researchers who examined the effect of psychological debriefing on emotional adaptation following a miscarriage found that the participants consistently reported "just having someone to talk to, someone who listened was helpful" (Lee et al., 1996, p. 56). Lee et al. (1996) cited previous research in which Slade and Willis found that over two-thirds of women would like some form of followup after their discharge. Unfortunately, many hospitals do not have a formal system for following up women who have had a miscarriage (Prettyman & Cordle, 1992). Thus, despite a strong awareness on the part of hospital staff that psychological sequelae of miscarriage are important issues, women tend to report high levels of dissatisfaction with the care and information provided to them (Friedman, 1989, as cited in Prettyman & Cordle, 1992; Reinharz, 1988). In addition to dissatisfaction with the medical team's response, women also find that partners, friends, and family members are uncomfortable talking about the miscarriage or stillbirth experience (Rajan & Oakley, 1993). Thus, many women feel stigmatized and silenced as they live the taboo of pregnancy loss.

Although stillbirth has been less well-studied, some general comments can be made regarding the emotional impact and the process of healing. The researchers who conducted one of the largest and most in-depth studies of the psychological, social, and somatic effects of stillbirth (DeFrain et al., 1990) concluded that women, partners, and family members are "permanently changed" following a stillbirth. Shock, blame, guilt, emotional hardship, irrational thoughts, and even feelings of momentary "craziness" are normative after a stillbirth (see also Woods & Esposito, 1987). Recovery is described as a "very, very slow process, much slower than people previously guessed," whereby it takes mothers and fathers (unfortunately, this study only included heterosexual couples) "an average of about three years to regain the level of happiness they felt before the death of the child" (DeFrain et al., 1990, p. 104). It should also be noted that recent advances in technology have changed the stillbirth experience dramatically in that "up until a few years ago many advanced fetal deaths occurred with little warning . . . with technological sophistication many if not most fetal deaths are predicted before delivery" (Kirkley-Best & VanDevere, 1986, p. 433). Technological advances mean that women may have to endure the agony of carrying a baby who is dead for weeks or even months. One woman in DeFrain et al.'s (1990) study who found out that the baby had died two and a half months before delivery stated, "I had time to adjust, but there are just no words to explain how it felt to walk around with a nonviable fetus" (p. 86).

IMPLICATIONS FOR THERAPY

Women who have experienced a pregnancy loss often come to therapy feeling isolated in their grief, frustrated and hurt by responses of partners, family, and friends, and mourning a future that is no longer possible in the way that they had once imagined. Thus, therapists need to be aware of the fact that many of their clients who have had a miscarriage or stillbirth have been dissatisfied with the lack of follow-up and/or with the specific responses (or lack thereof) of their heath care professionals. In light of this perceived lack of support, and based on the review of the research literature on the aftermath of perinatal loss, the following recommendations are made.

Help women identify the personal legacy of the loss. Meaning making is an idiosyncratic process; the diversity of responses that women have following pregnancy loss, and the difficulty researchers have had in identifying risk factors that can account for significant emotional distress, demonstrates just how individualized and nonformulaic the aftermath experience is. For example, although a stillbirth experience is devastating for nearly every mother (DeFrain et al., 1990), the research also demonstrates that therapists must avoid conflating gestational stage with increased distress. Both quantitative research and case study analysis suggest that pregnancy loss is a profound event that must be understood within the context of a woman's life history and within the specific meaning that the pregnancy and motherhood in general have for her (Reinharz, 1988; Swanson, 1999).

Appreciating the sociopolitical context in which the loss is embedded. Privileging the *personal* meanings of a woman's stillbirth or miscarriage experience need not make therapists lose sight of the *social* meanings of pregnancy loss. The epistemological framework that grounds feminist therapy encourages us to be highly attuned to the ways in which structural forces shape women's lives; we work hard at "deprivatizing distress" (Brown, 1994). To deprivatize distress and appreciate the sociopolitical context in which pregnancy loss is embedded means that therapists should understand the complex ways in which the medicalization of pregnancy and the subsequent "rhetoric of fetal endangerment" produces a cultural climate in which women *are* held responsible for fetal outcome (Markens et al., 1997). Hence, therapists must attend to how this cultural climate sustains grief and depression and fuels feelings of guilt and self-recrimination.

Understanding the aftermath as "disenfranchised grief." One of the most consistent findings in the research literature, that appears to be equally true for both miscarriage and stillbirth experience, is that the healing process is undermined by the lack of rituals for pregnancy loss, for they are losses that are not typically perceived as deaths to be mourned (Reinharz, 1988). Remembering the baby that was lost by having a funeral ceremony, a memorial service, a personalized grieving ritual, honoring anniversary dates of the loss or birth, and keeping mementos are all ways in which the grieving process can feel less disenfranchised (see Brin, this volume). This appears to be especially true for clients who have had a stillborn child; the literature suggests that seeing the stillborn baby and having a funeral are important parts of the grieving process. Also, it may be helpful to remind clients that contrary to the popularized notion of the grieving process, it is not typically experienced as phasic. That is, there has been a tendency to assume that grief progresses in discrete linear stages. However, the contributions of Kubler-Ross notwith-standing, research on the aftermath experiences of loss and traumas (see, for example, Cosgrove, 1988) suggests that a phasic model does not do justice to an individual's lived experience. Thus, it may be helpful for women to know that they are not "regressing" or "crazy" if they experience increased distress at various points, despite the fact they may indeed be "making progress" in therapy. Therefore, not only should therapists support women and their part-ners in their attempts to develop personalized rituals for grieving the loss, but therapists may have to counter some misperceptions about the grieving pro-cess–misperceptions that tend to sustain feelings of self-recrimination (e.g., "Why am I not over it yet?"). Stated most succinctly, resolution should not be equated with a simple return to a pre-loss level of functioning (Cosgrove, 1988).

The critical importance of social support. As previously noted, women who have experienced a miscarriage or stillbirth frequently report feeling hurt and disappointed by the responses (or lack thereof) made by partners, friends, hos-pital staff, and family members. DeFrain et al. (1990) summed this up well:

> Babies just do not die anymore. At least that's what most of us come to believe . . . it's not a topic of conversation when it does happen, or it is talked about in hushed tones . . . couple our discomfort as a society with the fact that fewer babies die today because of medical nutritional, public health advances, and a perfect setting for a conspiracy of silence is con-structed. (p. 90)

The conspiracy of silence can be overcome, and speech can heal broken community (Wertz, 1985), insofar as therapy becomes a place where a woman does not experience the social discomfort of the others to whom she tries to speak about her loss and pain. There are now a number of Internet support ser-vices available (see Appendix), and many women and their partners have found these sites very helpful. Indeed, finally having the opportunity to iden-tify and express powerful emotions, especially in the presence of supportive others, can be enormously powerful and healing. In this regard, it should be emphasized that heterosexist assumptions–and beliefs about who has the right to be a mother and thus whose loss "counts"–not only inform research agen-das, but these assumptions have also silenced the voices of poor, single, or les-bian mothers, and nontraditional couples who experience pregnancy loss. Feminist therapists are, of course, sensitive to these assumptions and their im-pact; however, our sensitivity must translate into concrete action. As therapists we can actively reach out to those women who might need to talk about their loss, but have not had the opportunity to do so. (For example, therapists could work collaboratively with local shelters to provide direct services to women in shelters who have experienced pregnancy loss, or to train the staff to be supportive.)

Reflectively attending to one's countertransference issues. It is critically important for therapists to be aware that pregnancy loss may engender intense emotional responses and thus to be vigilantly on guard for the ways in which countertransference issues will impact on the therapeutic relationship. Therapists must "be personally able to bear empathically the painful affects without deflecting or avoiding that intensity . . . [and their] personal life [must not be] in crisis regarding childbearing issues" (Elkin, 1990, pp. 605-606). However, it should not be assumed that it is only those therapists who have struggled with fertility or pregnancy loss issues who will be vulnerable to having countertransference issues. Unfortunately, countertransference is often interpreted quite narrowly–as an unconscious reaction to a client that is based on the therapist's *personal* history and "baggage." Feminist therapists reject this narrow definition and instead recognize that countertransference is an inevitable, but valuable, part of any therapeutic relationship; it is source of information about the therapist, the client, the therapeutic relationship, and the *social* myths that both the therapist and client have internalized. For example, all therapists, even those who identify strongly as feminists, have internalized some of the sexist and blaming discourses related to the role of maternal responsibility for pregnancy outcome. Thus, all clinicians must remain open to identifying and analyzing the ways in which these social myths impact on their therapy.

CONCLUSION

Women who have experienced a pregnancy loss have been underserved. Indeed, researchers and clinicians have much to learn about coping from women who have experienced miscarriages and stillbirths, for the vocabulary of the medical model not only fails to capture their lived experience, but it also sustains a focus on pathology. Therefore, it can not be emphasized enough how important it is to create a space where women have the opportunity to identify and "own" the ways in which they have survived their loss and have created meaning out of it. Honoring women's sense-making, appreciating both traditional and nontraditional coping strategies, and exploring resilience should be an integral part of the therapeutic process. If we are to bear witness to our clients' power (Brown, 1994) and resilience, then we must challenge the epistemological framework of our biomedical discourse. In so doing, we will be serving the needs of women who have experienced pregnancy loss, as well as contributing to the development of a transformative therapeutic approach–one that privileges the sociopolitical context in which women interpret and give meaning to their experience of loss.

NOTES

1. All of the estimates given are for the U.S.
2. An important exception is Markens, Browner, and Press (1997).
3. However, it is important to note that Black and Hispanic women are clearly at greater risk for pregnancy loss than White women (National Center for Health Statistics, 2000).

REFERENCES

Armstrong, E. M. (2000). Lessons in control: Prenatal education in the hospital. *Social Problems, 47*, 583-605.

Beil, E. R. (1992). Miscarriage: The influence of selected variables on impact. *Women & Therapy, 12* (1), 161-173.

Borg, S., & Lasker, J. N. (1989). *When pregnancy fails: Families coping with miscarriage, ectopic pregnancy, stillbirth, and infant death.* New York: Bantam.

Brin, D. (2004). The use of rituals in grieving for a miscarriage or stillbirth. *Women & Therapy, 27*(3/4), 123-132.

Brown, L. S. (1994). *Subversive dialogues: Theory in feminist therapy.* New York: Basic Books.

Burr, V. (1995). *An introduction to social constructionism.* Florence, KY: Taylor & Francis/Routledge.

Cecil, R. (1994). Miscarriage: Women's views of care. *Journal of Reproductive and Infant Psychology, 12*, 21-29.

Chung, P. H., & Yeko, T. R. (1996). Recurrent miscarriage: Causes and management. *Hospital Practice, 31*, 157-164.

Condon, J. T. (1986). Management of established pathological grief reaction after stillbirth. *American Journal of Psychiatry, 143*, 987-992.

Cosgrove, L. (1988, March). *Victims' responses to sexual assault.* Paper presented at the annual meeting of the Association for Women in Psychology. Bethesda, MD.

Cosgrove, L. (2000). Crying out loud: Understanding women's emotional distress as both lived experience and social construction. *Feminism & Psychology, 10*, 247-267.

Cosgrove, L., & Riddle, B. (2003). Constructions of femininity and experiences of menstrual distress. *Women & Health, 38*, 39-60.

DeFrain, J. (1991). Learning about grief from normal families: SIDS, stillbirth, and miscarriage. *Journal of Marital and Family Therapy, 17*, 215-232.

DeFrain, J., Martens, L., Stork, J., & Stork, W. (1990). The psychological and social effects of a stillbirth on surviving family members. *Omega: Journal of Death and Dying, 22*, 83-110.

Doka, K. J. (1989). *Disenfranchised grief: Recognizing hidden sorrow.* Lexington, MA: Lexington Books/D.C. Heath.

Dunbar, H. F. (1954). *Emotions and bodily changes* (4th ed.). New York: Columbia.

Elkin, E. F. (1990). When a patient miscarries: Implications for treatment. *Psychotherapy, 27*, 600-606.

Fausto-Sterling, A. (2000). *Myths of gender: Biological theories about women and men.* New York: Basic Books.

Fine, M. (1992). *Disruptive voices: The possibilities of feminist research.* Ann Arbor, MI: University of Michigan Press.

Friedman, T., & Gath, D. (1989). The psychiatric consequences of spontaneous abortion. *British Journal of Psychiatry, 155*, 810-813.

Gardner, C. B. (1995). Learning for two: A study in the rhetoric of pregnancy practices. *Perspectives on Social Problems, 7*, 29-51.

Gergen, K. J. (1994). *Realities and relationships: Soundings in social construction.* Cambridge, MA: Harvard University Press.

Glazer, E. S. (1997). Miscarriage and its aftermath. In S. R. Leiblum (Ed.), *Infertility: Psychological issues and counseling strategies* (pp. 230-245). New York: Wiley.

Harding, J. (1998). *Sex acts practices of femininity and masculinity.* London: Sage.

Hertz, D. G. (1973). Rejection of motherhood: A psychosomatic appraisal of habitual abortion. *Psychosomatics, 14*, 241-244.

Janssen, H. J., Cuisiner, M. C., de Graauw, K. P., & Hoogduin, K. A. (1997). A prospective study of risk factors predicting grief intensity following pregnancy loss. *Archives of General Psychiatry, 54*, 56-61.

Kirkley-Best, E., & Kellner, K. R. (1982). The forgotten grief: A review of the psychology of stillbirth. *American Journal of Orthopsychiatry, 52*, 420-429.

Kirkley-Best, E., & VanDevere, C. (1986). The hidden family grief: An overview of grief in the family following perinatal death. *International Journal of Family Psychiatry, 7*, 419-437.

Lee, C., Slade, P., & Lygo, V. (1996). The influence of psychological debriefing on emotional adaptation in women following early miscarriage: A preliminary study. *British Journal of Medical Psychology, 69*, 47-58.

Leppert, P. C., & Pahlka, B. S. (1984). Grieving characteristics after spontaneous abortion: A management approach. *Obstetrics and Gynecology, 64*, 119-122.

Markens, S., Browner, C. H., & Press, N. (1997). Feeding the fetus: On interrogating the notion of maternal-fetal conflict. *Feminist Studies, 23*, 351-372.

Martin, E. (1987). *The women in the body: A cultural analysis of reproduction.* Boston: Beacon Press.

Moulder, C. (1994). Towards a preliminary framework for understanding pregnancy loss. *Journal of Reproductive and Infant Psychology, 12*, 65-67.

Murray, J., & Callan, J. (1988). Predicting adjustment to perinatal death. *British Journal of Medical Psychology, 61*, 237-244.

National Center for Health Statistics. (2000). *Trends in pregnancy and pregnancy rates by outcome: Estimates for the United States 1976-96, 21* (DHHS Publication No. PHS 2000-1934). Washington, DC: U.S. Government Printing Office.

Peppers, I., & Knapp, R. (1980). *Motherhood and mourning: Perinatal death.* New York: Praeger.

Petchesky, R. (1987). Fetal images: The power of the visual culture in the politics of reproduction. *Feminist Studies, 13,* 263-292.

Prettyman, R. J., & Cordle, C. (1992). Psychological aspects of miscarriage: Attitudes of the primary health care team. *British Journal of General Practice, 42,* 97-99.

Prettyman, R. J., Cordle, C. J., & Cook, G. D. (1993). A three-month follow-up of psychological morbidity after early miscarriage. *British Journal of Medical Psychology, 66,* 363-372.

Rajan, L., & Oakley, A. (1993). No pills for heartache: The importance of social support for women who suffer pregnancy loss. *Journal of Reproductive and Infant Psychology, 11,* 75-87.

Reinharz, S. (1988). What's missing in miscarriage? *Journal of Community Psychology, 16,* 84-103.

Shapiro, C. H. (1993). *When part of the self is lost: Helping clients heal after sexual and reproductive losses.* San Francisco: Jossey-Bass.

Slade, P. (1994). Predicting the psychological impact of miscarriage. *Journal of Reproductive and Infant Psychology, 12,* 5-16.

Smart, C. (1992). (Ed.). *Regulating womanhood. Historical essays on marriage, motherhood and sexuality.* New York: Routledge.

Squier, R., & Dunbar, F. (1946). Emotional factors in the course of pregnancy. *Psychosomatic Medicine, 8,* 161-175.

Swanson, K. M. (1999). Effects of caring, measurement, and time on miscarriage impact and women's well-being. *Nursing Research, 48,* 288-298.

Thapar, A. K., & Thapar, A. (1992). Psychological sequelae of miscarriage: A controlled study using the general health questionnaire and the hospital anxiety and depression scale. *British Journal of General Practice, 42,* 94-96.

Ussher, J. (1996). Premenstrual syndrome: Reconciling disciplinary divides through the adoption of a material-discursive epistemological standpoint. *Annual Review of Sex Research, 7,* 218-251.

Weil, R. J., & Tupper, C. (1960). Personality, life situation, and communication: A study of habitual abortion. *Psychosomatic Medicine, 22,* 448-455.

Wertz, F. (1985). Method and findings in a phenomenological psychological study of a complex life event: Being criminally victimized. In A. Giorgi (Ed.), *Phenomenology and psychological research* (pp. 155-216). Pittsburgh: Duquesne University Press.

Wilcox, A. J., Weinberg, C. R., O'Connor, J. F., Baird, D. D., Schlatterer, J. P., Canfield, R. E., Armstrong, E. G., & Nisula, B. C. (1988). Incidence of early pregnancy loss. *New England Journal of Medicine, 319,* 189-194.

Woods, J. R., & Esposito, J. L. (Eds.). (1987). *Pregnancy loss: Medical therapeutics and practical considerations.* Baltimore: Williams & Wilkins.

Zita, J. N. (1988). The premenstrual syndrome: "Dis-easing" the female cycle. *Hypatia, 3,* 157-168.

APPENDIX

Organizations and Web Sites

Compassionate Friends: A national nonprofit organization that provides information and support following the death of an infant or child. There is no religious affiliation and no membership dues. <www.compassionatefriends.org>

H.A.N.D. (Helping After Neonatal Death) offers support and information following a miscarriage, stillbirth, or newborn's death. The following services are offered: resource library, phone support, peer support groups, in-service programs for heath providers. P.O. Box 371, Los Gatos, CA 95031; (408) 732-3228

StillFathers: A resource for fathers who have experienced stillbirth, infant death, or miscarriage. <www.stillfathers.org>

WiSSP (Wisconsin Stillbirth Service Program): A community-based, university-supported model for the investigation of causes of stillbirth. WiSSP serves families and professionals in Wisconsin and throughout the world by providing support resources, educational material, and scientific and medical data to families and medical personnel. <www.wisc/edu/wissp/wisco.htm/>

The Use of Rituals in Grieving for a Miscarriage or Stillbirth

Deborah J. Brin

SUMMARY. Preparation for their changing roles in family and society, as well as readying their intimate space for the arrival of an infant, totally engage expectant parents. Miscarriage or stillbirth may bring on a grief storm that strips away many tender roots and branches of new life in the community that the parents have been nurturing. Creation and participation in a grief ritual can bring the grieving parents to a healing resolution. This article describes the healing efficacy of ritual, its elements, and how a compassionate therapist can create one in collaboration with grieving clients. *[Article copies available for a fee from The Haworth Document Delivery Service: 1-800-HAWORTH. E-mail address: <docdelivery@haworthpress.com> Website:*

Deborah J. Brin, MA, MAHL, was ordained as a rabbi in 1985, and has served as a pastoral counselor in a variety of rabbinic positions, including congregational leadership and institutional chaplaincy. She is currently Associate Chaplain at Grinnell College. Her account of leading a women's prayer ritual at the Western Wall in Jerusalem was recently published in *Women of the Wall: Claiming Sacred Ground at Judaism's Holy Site.*

Address correspondence to: Rabbi Deborah J. Brin, 602 11th Ave., Grinnell, IA 50112 (E-mail: brin@grinnell.edu).

Author note: I would like to thank all of those who have invited me into their lives to ritualize their healing process and to be present with them in times of joy as well as crisis; Lynn (Yael) McKeever; the members of B'not Esh, a Jewish feminist community; Rebecca Alpert and Linda Holtzman; and Aviva Goldberg, for sharing thoughts and themes from her unpublished dissertation *Awakening Deborah: A Feminist Analysis of Contemporary Jewish Renewal Liturgy, Ritual and Theology.*

[Haworth co-indexing entry note]: "The Use of Rituals in Grieving for a Miscarriage or Stillbirth." Brin, Deborah J. Co-published simultaneously in *Women & Therapy* (The Haworth Press, Inc.) Vol. 27, No. 3/4, 2004, pp. 123-132; and: *From Menarche to Menopause: The Female Body in Feminist Therapy* (ed: Joan C. Chrisler) The Haworth Press, Inc., 2004, pp. 123-132. Single or multiple copies of this article are available for a fee from The Haworth Document Delivery Service [1-800-HAWORTH, 9:00 a.m. - 5:00 p.m. (EST). E-mail address: docdelivery@haworthpress.com].

KEYWORDS. Rituals for healing, miscarriage, stillbirth, grief for death of an infant, Jewish perspectives on grief, Judaism and women

The powerful energy of ritual helps parents heal from pregnancy loss by acknowledging the traumatic event, drawing to them the healing presence of their friends and family, and providing the comfort of tradition. Ritual functions to mark a liminal moment of transition that can begin, promote, or accelerate emotional and spiritual healing. As a rabbi with graduate training in counseling, I have had the privilege of being invited into the deep spaces of grief and have heard parents' pain. I share this terrain with therapists and other emotional healers. My approach has been to create healing rituals that are personally significant for the parents and, at the same time, universally symbolic and meaningful, so that all who wish to lend their love and support to the anguished mother and father can feel the relief of actually "doing something" to help.

In my rabbinate, I have created healing rituals for domestic violence, incest, and rape, as well as ceremonial expressions of community grief for public tragedies such as September 11th and community-wide trauma over the violent death of young college students. I think of ritual as the creation of an "elongated moment" that separates the past from the future and acknowledges the life force that moves through us in times of unexpected and unwelcome change.

Ritual is usually associated with religion. For religious persons, participation in traditional rituals acknowledges universal life cycle events, ameliorates pain, amplifies joy, and enhances connection with the community. However, most of the traditional religions are shackled with andocentric worldviews that discount or ignore women's experiences as human beings in a female embodiment. Few have adapted to the changes in consciousness brought about by the medical technology of our age, where women can become pregnant through artificial insemination and in-vitro techniques, and where parents plan pregnancies and have mutual experiences (via sonograms and ultrasounds) with their children even before they are born. These technologies have emerged within a social and cultural context where women need and expect public recognition of their personal experiences.

The purpose of this article, however, is not to discuss how religion can adapt to the needs of contemporary society. Here I address the reality that, at least partly because religions provide no formal rituals for dealing with many of the traumas of modern life, individuals find themselves in psychotherapy trying to contend with their feelings of loss, isolation, powerlessness, and fear of trying again. Among Jews with whom I have worked, such feelings are compounded by the anger born of having their needs discounted by the elders in the community and the humiliation of having God's will interpreted to them in an anti-feminist, even misogynistic, pronouncement. In the aftermath of people's frustrated search for traditional ritual and rejection by the established interpreters of tradition, psychotherapy clients can find great solace in feeling empowered to create their own rituals.

Our lives are actually filled with rituals, even though we may not recognize them as such. Whenever we anticipate a transitional moment, prepare for it, and mark it with concrete symbolism that is consciously repetitive of similar transitions in our own lives with others, we are participating in ritual. It could be telling a child a bedtime story, doing "the wave" at a baseball game, or moving the tassel to the other side of the mortarboard as we walk off the stage with our diplomas. Thus, creating ritual is not an extraordinary endeavor. The basic process of creating ritual is part of our continual search for meaning, and we do it all the time by repeating the stories we tell, elevating certain objects to having symbolic meanings, and associating songs and melodies with regular actions or special events.

The healing efficacy of the rituals women and couples create around the experiences of miscarriage, stillbirth, or death of an infant begins with the creative process of focusing their intentions and searching for the elements that bring meaning and significance to the flow of events. Many such rituals include friends and family members as participants or witnesses who deliver meaningful content and purpose into the external, social network that surrounds the mourners. Among the benefits of externalizing grief and joy through ritual is asking for acknowledgement of what has transpired and support for the process of letting go and moving on.

Feminists say that the personal is the political. Jewish feminists have for the last three decades declared that the stories of our lives are sacred texts.[1] The subjective is an artery from the universal, and ritual completes the flow of consciousness from and through our own lives to the life of our communities.

In the academic study of religion, the methodology of studying the power of religion through the subjective experience of a participant is called "ethno hermeneutics." This phrase acknowledges that, on the one hand, the report of one person's story is not objective proof of the efficacy of the function of ritual, and, on the other hand, that personal experience and observations are valid and informative data (personal communication, Aviva Goldberg, January 2002). In this spirit, I would like to describe a healing ritual that I helped to create for a bereaved couple.

A STORY OF HEALING THROUGH RITUAL

The first time that I was privileged to assist a couple with unfinished grief about a stillbirth was in Toronto, Canada, in 1987. I was a rookie rabbi, serving my first pulpit, when I was approached after services one day by a new congregant. She briefly explained that she and her husband would like to meet with me to discuss creating a ritual to help them grieve their stillborn daughter. I was prepared to be helpful because one of the intentions of my rabbinate was to make Jewish tradition more transparent and accessible so that the psychological needs of congregants could be met. However, I didn't know much about the emotional and spiritual impact of a stillbirth. We agreed to begin our conversations later that week at their home, where it would be easy for them to talk while taking care of Daniel, their one-year-old son. Often a member of the clergy has a relationship with congregants before they go into mourning, but Jane, Harold, and I were getting to know each other for the first time. They told me the story of their daughter, whom they had affectionately named "Junior" while she was still alive in utero. Junior had been stillborn two winters before.

From my feminist perspective, I thought of pregnancy loss as a woman's issue and was surprised at the idea that I would be meeting with both Jane and Harold. They made it a point to express to me how important it was for both of them to acknowledge their feelings. Over and over again, Harold had been made invisible after the event of the stillbirth of his daughter. Other people treated him as though he was a bystander, that it hadn't really happened to him, too, and that he hadn't had anything to lose or grieve. This treatment reinforced all of the stereotypes that men are supposed to be strong and not show any emotions.

Through their still-palpable pain and gentle conversational manner, they taught me what I needed to know in order to be able to help. I learned about the contours of their grief and the frustrations of their efforts to deal with it. They both said, in different ways, that they had lost not only the person of their first child, but they had lost their dreams of becoming parents and their plans to become a family. They had spent months eagerly preparing, making space in their lives and in their home for the new baby. Then came the shock and grief of discovering that the baby girl had died in the womb.

After the difficult decisions about birthing a dead baby, and the coolness of the medical staff during the actual process, Jane and Harold then had to face decisions about the disposition of the small corpse. They sought the advice of a rabbi who explained the procedure for burial and who told them not to go themselves to the cemetery but to "go home and make another baby." They did go to the cemetery. A makeshift and perfunctory burial was carried out by an obliging but inexperienced funeral director. It was a bleak and blustery Canadian winter day, and the bereft parents were physically miserable and exhausted. The funeral director marked the grave with a small metallic stake that had Junior's name in dyno-tape . . . no headstone, prayers, songs, or ritual. No community of mourners or witnesses to the event. No meal waiting at home, prepared by loving hands to feed their emptiness. They felt abandoned and rejected by the Jewish community, and their feelings were invalidated and invisible.

They spoke of how they had managed to work through some of their grief both separately and together, but of how much they still wanted to experience healing and gain some sense of closure on the event. Even though it had been over two years since Junior had died, they wanted a funeral ritual, they wanted it to be Jewish, they wanted it to be personal, and they needed to feel the acceptance, support, and understanding of the Jewish community. My willingness to assist them with planning the ritual gave them the "official sanction" they needed.

Some of the necessary elements of the ritual were clear because Jane and Harold knew that they wanted symbols from Jewish tradition. They also felt certainty that the ceremony should be simple and that it should take place at the site of the original burial. They wanted to be able to talk to Junior and not be made to feel self-conscious or shamed in any way. I would be the only other person present, serving a dual role as officiant and as a representative of the Jewish community.

We agreed that the spring would be a good time to go to the cemetery, that Jane and Harold would each write something that they would read aloud about their hopes and dreams of becoming parents, of the grief they experienced when Junior died, and of how they have coped since her death. When they finished reading their "letters to Junior," I would sing the traditional funeral prayer "El Maleh Rachamim" and then lead them in the mourner's prayer, the "kaddish."

When the appointed day arrived, I realized that a key element was missing from the plan–we needed to dig in the earth. We needed to "bury" something. I grabbed a couple of trowels, and on my drive to meet Jane and Harold, I stopped at a gardening store. I gazed perplexed at all of the flowers. This was a last minute addition and I hadn't consulted with them, so I didn't have any idea of what kind of plant would be the most appropriate. I chose some flowers that looked to me like tiny pansies. When I arrived at their apartment prior to going to the cemetery, I told them of my idea and showed them the plants. Jane was delighted. It turns out that the plants are called "Johnny jump ups," and they were her favorite.

At the cemetery, Jane led us to the place were she believed that Junior had been buried. The flimsy metal marker had long since disappeared. This, alone, was a reawakening of the rawness of the unfinished grief. We settled on a spot, and began our ritual. At the end, Jane and Harold planted the flowers, and then we rested together in silence. After a time, they began to talk about the future, their son, and their hope for more children. After the ceremony, they went to the home of some friends who had watched Daniel for them, and they had a "mourners' meal" together.

Fourteen years later, I happened to be in Toronto and had the opportunity to visit with Jane (Harold wasn't able to join us) and again to meet their son, Daniel then 15.[2] It was good to see Daniel and to hear how the family was doing. During this visit, Jane reaffirmed to me that the ultimate function of the ritual we had created was for closure on their unfinished grief. She also let me know that it had worked. She had had two more miscarriages and another stillbirth subsequent to my departure from Toronto. So much pain and grief! She and Harold had often assisted others through the difficult experiences of pregnancy loss and stillbirth. They share their own experiences, listen to those of the other couples, and, when the time is right, encourage them to create their own rituals. Jane told me that 75% of couples that go through a stillbirth end up divorcing. She and Harold had beaten the odds. Because of her deeply felt need to be of service to people who become cut off by their circumstances, Jane had enrolled in graduate school in social work and was embarking on a career of helping others to cope with miscarriages, stillbirths, and infant death.

CREATING RITUAL

Every ritual will be unique to the person or people who are creating it. It provides an opportunity to address people's deep need to express themselves. Some may find the term "ritual" to be a roadblock, and changing the name may help to get the energy flowing. Call it an "event" or "ceremony" or even a "party." The gathering of people and energy is the goal.

Rituals have a focus and a flow. Every ritual occurs in time at a particular moment and makes a distinction between that which came before and the hopes, dreams, and potential that reside in the unknown future. Regardless of when the death occurred, the awareness during a ritual must be on the "now." Tremendous energy can be mobilized and focused on the central intention if it is centered in the here and now.

The first answer that needs to emerge from a dialogic process with a client is, simply, what is the central intention of the ritual? As in other creative processes, there are many variables, many possibilities, and many questions to be addressed. Therapists will probably already know a lot about the client's healing process, but it is important nevertheless to formulate simple questions about who the significant people are, in what stage they are in their grief process, what else has happened in their lives since the event of the miscarriage or stillbirth, and how easy or difficult it is for them to empower themselves to engage in the creation of a ritual. The therapist's questions should engage the client in envisioning the results of the process and the way things will be different after the ritual or ceremony. After the goals are clear, the "how" of making it happen will be easier to determine. For instance, Jane and Harold articulated that they needed to finish their grieving for Junior and they needed not only to have Jewish elements but also the presence of an understanding rabbi to repair the damage done by the lack of official recognition at the time of the stillbirth. The rest of the planning flowed from knowing what they needed.

The ability to determine the central intention of the ritual is facilitated by clinical understandings of the grief process. Knowing where a client (and perhaps her spouse/partner) is on the continuum of grief will clarify the conversations about the ritual and, to some extent, determine the selection of ritual elements for the ceremony. Perhaps the client and her partner/spouse have struggled with experiences of multiple miscarriages and, because of their grief work, are now ready to begin the process of adoption. Such plans are important "next chapters" in their story and good foci for the imagination. They have had experiences that they want to let go of completely so that they can step fresh and invigorated into a new phase of their lives. They want to mobilize their energy and focus it in a new direction. Perhaps the ceremony for hopeful parents who are turning toward adoption could be a tree planting picnic/party in their backyard. The tree would be a memorial to the unborn ones, and the picnic would celebrate their readiness wholeheartedly to become adoptive parents.

Another very different ritual could focus on renewing hope of birthing a healthy child. Perhaps the woman who has experienced a miscarriage or multiple miscarriages wants to continue to try to carry a pregnancy to term. She may decide that what she needs is for her women friends and relatives to gather in a private and safe place and focus their energy, good wishes, and blessings on her body. Maybe they would give her massages, paint her toenails, draw on her body with henna or body paint, or place their hands on her belly and give her blessings. Perhaps they will conclude by eating food that they have prepared for her that has fruit as its essential ingredient. Why fruit? In many cultures it is symbolic of fertility because it holds its seeds within itself.

Rituals are creative uses of the medium of time. Think of the ritual as an elongated moment, a moment squeezed for all it is worth to make a memorable distinction between what came before and what comes after. Like a symphony or theatrical play, this elongated moment has a specific setting/place and a definite beginning, middle, and end.

The central focus of the event, the turning point, are the words or gestures that communicate the ritual intent. But intention determines far more than what is said and done in the middle of the ceremony. What will happen in the elongated moment determines where it will take place, who the participants are, the tone and feel of the event, how long it will last, whether it is private or public, and how formal or informal it will be. Much of the preparation streams into the "beginning" of the ritual, and it is ideal to be able to create concrete benchmarks to the specific point in time that is the beginning of the ritual. The beginning is a physical act of creating community such as the joining of voices in song or the touching of hands in a circle. Even a private ritual should define who is present, including the spirits or memories of the deceased. It is the bringing of emotion and thought into the realm of the senses that makes ritual an art form. Seeing, hearing, and touching all give spatial veracity to the marking of time in the elongated moment. The end of the ritual is the physical act of separation. It can be symbolized by flowing water, burning fire, or turning earth, and it may be marked by the formality of dispersing the gathering in a recessional or dance.

Once all of these questions have been discussed and the ritual itself has begun to emerge, it can be useful to plot it out on paper. Write down the basic outline, so that the stages and elements are all clear. What are the beginning, the middle, and the end? Indicate who will speak or act during a given section of the ritual and what "props" they will need. If it is a very simple ritual, it may be sufficient to tell friends and family members to meet in the backyard at a certain time, plant a tree together, and then have a picnic. If it is more complex, it can be important to have lists of all of the "props." If candles are an element of the ceremony, someone needs to bring matches. If wine will be used, a corkscrew needs to be brought so that the bottle can be opened. When guests will be invited to sing along, song sheets can be very helpful.

It is helpful to "frame" the ritual activity in ordinary time. To distinguish the moment of beginning, there can be deliberate placement of pictures or cards in a lobby or entering room to encourage people to chat and engage in small talk. The mourners' meal that follows a ceremony, for example, should not be formal and sanctimonious but free-flowing and casual.

CONCLUSION

There are some ethical and practical challenges to the therapist who is assisting a client in the creation of a public or shared event. First of all, because of the confidential, private nature of the counseling relationship, it may be awkward to include essential people in the planning conversations. As Jane and Harold pointed out, a ritual for the loss of a child is a process for parents to engage in together to heal their own relationship. If only one of the parents is a client and the co-parenting relationship is intact, it is important to address the need to include the absent parent. Second, because the efficacy of the ritual for most people is the ability to be swept up in it and not be "in charge," an officiator, such as a clergyperson or a friend who plays the role of "ritual m.c.," is an essential element. For a therapist to step outside the therapeutic relationship to take up this role is often inadvisable. However, planning the ritual without the wherewithal to implement the plan may also be a disservice. These are dilemmas for the therapist and the clients to work through. I can assure you, though, that there are many sensitive and proactive clergypersons on the scene today, and many of them are eager to be of service in this way.

NOTES

1. See Rabbi Sue Levi Elwell's MA thesis *Text and Transformation: Towards a Theology of Integrity,* especially Chapter 2: "Our lives as texts."
2. April 2002.

REFERENCE

Elwell, S. L. (1986). *Text & transformation: Towards a theology of integrity.* Unpublished MA thesis, Hebrew Union College-Jewish Institute of Religion, Cincinnati, OH.

RESOURCES

Krohn, I., Moffitt, P-l., & Wilkins, I. A. (2000). *A silent sorrow.* New York: Routledge. This book is a solid resource book for those who have suffered from pregnancy loss. Its chapters on grief and the differences between grieving mothers and grieving fathers, as well as the chapter on finding solace in religion are excellent.

Stinson, K. M., Lasker, J. L., Lohmann, J., & Toedter, L. J. (1992). Parents' grief following pregnancy loss: A comparison of mothers and fathers. *Family Relations, Journal of Applied Family and Child Studies, 41,* 218-223. This article focuses on gender differences in grieving a pregnancy loss and the tension caused by this incongruence.

Callan, V. J., & Murray, J. (1989). The role of therapists in helping couples cope with stillbirth and newborn death. *Family Relations: Journal of Applied Family and Child Studies, 38,* 248-253. This article articulates the need for family therapists to assist a couple in grieving a stillborn child and acknowledges that resolution of that grief may not occur before 2 years have passed.

Condon, J. (1986). Management of established pathological grief reaction after Stillbirth. *American Journal of Psychiatry, 143,* 987-992. This article describes the unique aspects to the grief for a stillborn child due to the "unique psychobiological climate in which the loss occurs."

Weintraub, S. Y. (Ed.). (1994). *Healing of soul, healing of body: Spiritual leaders unfold the strength and solace in Psalms.* Woodstock, VT: Jewish Lights Publishing. Selected psalms are translated and commented on by contemporary rabbis who focus on making the psalms accessible and meaningful to those engaged in the spiritual task of healing.

Dossey, L. (1996). *Prayer is good medicine.* San Francisco: Harper. This popular book deals with the results of the new scientific studies that show that prayer has a positive impact on healing. An easy read, it may be helpful for those who have rejected religion. Dossey does point out that prayer and the act of praying are not the sole property of organized religion.

Brin, D. J., & Sharkey, L. (1992). Jewish women creating ritual. *Fireweed, 35,* 70-73. This article describes the traditional Jewish life cycle ceremonies, their lacunae, and a personal perspective on the story of the ritual for Junior.

Umansky, E. M., & Ashton, D. (Eds). (1992). *Four centuries of Jewish women's spirituality: A sourcebook.* Boston: Beacon Press. There are a wide variety of Jewish women's voices and experiences throughout the centuries represented in this groundbreaking volume. The following selections may be of particular interest:

Healing after a miscarriage, a poem by Merle Feld, *The womb and the word: A fertility ritual for Hannah*, by Penina V. Adelman, *Mikvah ceremony for Laura*, by Laura Levitt and Sue Ann Waserman.

Starhawk. (1979). *The spiral dance: A rebirth of the ancient religion of the Great Goddess*. New York: Harper & Row. This book describes how to create rituals and the power and energy that inheres in them. It also teaches about sacred space and the worldview of pagan cultures, Goddess worshippers, and those who practice witchcraft.

Mykoff, M., & Mizrahi, S. C. (1999). *The gentle weapon: Prayers for everyday and not-so-everyday moments by the Rebbe Nachman of Breslov*. Woodstock, VT: Jewish Lights Publishing. This small book has 95 prayers/poems, useable by everyone, no matter what their background, that are adapted from prayers written by Reb Nachman, a Chassidic master (1772-1810).

Schnur, S., & Solomon, D. (1990/5750). Into the future with rituals from our past. *Lillith Magazine*, *15* (30), 19-23. This article describes two new Jewish rituals, one for a divorce and one after a miscarriage and includes a comment by anthropologist Riv-Ellen Prell.

Adelman, P. V. (1989/5749). A ritual for miscarriage. *The Reconstructionist*, *54* (4). In this groundbreaking article, Penina describes a ritual that she and her husband created after her miscarriage. The audacity to create a ritual of their own gave others the courage to create ritual for themselves as well.

Wiener, S. (1993). How do you mourn for a miscarriage or for a child's death during the first month? *Moment Magazine*, pp. 22-23. In this article, Rabbi Wiener suggests a model for creating a meaningful commemoration.

Orenstein, D. (Ed.). (1994). *Lifecycles: Jewish women on life passages and personal milestones*, *V.I.* Woodstock, NY: Jewish Lights Publishing. Of special interest here is the "prayer after a miscarriage or stillbirth" by Sandy Eisenberg Sasso. Also, see the afterword on how to create ritual by Rabbi Debra Orenstein.

Brin, D. J. (2003). Against the wall. In P. Chesler & R. Haut (Eds.), *Women of the wall: Claiming sacred ground at Judaism's holy site* (pp. 215-221). Woodstock, NY: Jewish Lights Publishing.

Psychological Issues in Childbirth: Potential Roles for Psychotherapists

Ingrid Johnston-Robledo
Jessica Barnack

SUMMARY. Despite the myriad psychosocial aspects of childbirth, psychologists have not contributed extensively to the childbirth literature nor are they identified as a resource for women who are either anticipating or adjusting after an inherently challenging life event. The purpose of this article is to review the current literature on psychosocial aspects of birthing to identify a variety of issues that would be of relevance to psychotherapists. We discuss both normative issues such as women's fears or concerns about giving birth as well as clinical issues such as traumatic birth experiences and complications for women with psychological disorders. Finally, we provide specific suggestions for practitioners so that they are better able to work with women and their partners during this pivotal time in their lives. We argue that psychotherapists are in an ideal position to provide women, particularly those at risk

Ingrid Johnston-Robledo, PhD, is Assistant Professor in the Psychology Department at State University of New York, College at Fredonia where she teaches courses in the Psychology of Women, Human Sexuality, and Women's Health. Her research interests concern women's experiences with childbirth, postpartum adjustment, and breastfeeding. Jessica Barnack graduated from the State University of New York with a bachelor's degree in Psychology. She is currently a graduate student at Connecticut College.

Address correspondence to: Ingrid Johnston-Robledo, PhD, Department of Psychology, State University of New York, College at Fredonia, Fredonia, NY 14063.

[Haworth co-indexing entry note]: "Psychological Issues in Childbirth: Potential Roles for Psychotherapists." Johnston-Robledo, Ingrid, and Jessica Barnack. Co-published simultaneously in *Women & Therapy* (The Haworth Press, Inc.) Vol. 27, No. 3/4, 2004, pp. 133-150; and: *From Menarche to Menopause: The Female Body in Feminist Therapy* (ed: Joan C. Chrisler) The Haworth Press, Inc., 2004, pp. 133-150. Single or multiple copies of this article are available for a fee from The Haworth Document Delivery Service [1-800-HAWORTH, 9:00 a.m. - 5:00 p.m. (EST). E-mail address: docdelivery@haworthpress.com].

http://www.haworthpress.com/store/product.asp?sku=J015
10.1300/J015v27n03_10

for adverse outcomes, with the support and skills necessary to prepare for, cope during, and adjust after the challenge of giving birth. *[Article copies available for a fee from The Haworth Document Delivery Service: 1-800-HAWORTH. E-mail address: <docdelivery@haworthpress.com> Website: <http://www.HaworthPress.com> © 2004 by The Haworth Press, Inc. All rights reserved.]*

KEYWORDS. Psychotherapists, pregnancy, birthing, traumatic birth, PTSD

Although childbirth may be regarded as challenging or even as a crisis to be managed, it is generally considered a normative event. As such, psychotherapists are rarely utilized by women during pregnancy or the postpartum period solely for purposes of preparing for or processing the event. However, researchers are beginning to examine relatively normative aspects of birthing that could potentially lead to adverse psychological outcomes, and some may warrant clinical intervention. These include fears about childbirth (Melender & Lauri, 1999), concerns about labor (Fowles, 1998), uncaring interactions with providers (Halldorsdottir & Karlsdottir, 1996), and obstetrical interventions (DiMatteo et al., 1996; Green, Coupland, & Kitzinger, 1990).

A serious clinical issue associated with birthing is an acute stress reaction or posttraumatic stress disorder (PTSD) as a result of a traumatic childbirth (Creedy, Shochet, & Horsfall, 2000; Wijma, Soderquist, & Wijma, 1997). Women who have a history of trauma, such as childhood sexual abuse, may find birthing especially challenging or traumatizing (Jacobs, 1992; Rhodes & Hutchinson, 1994). Women who have been diagnosed with schizophrenia, depression, or eating disorders also have unique needs and may experience birthing complications that a therapist could help address or prevent (Miller, 2001; Miller & Shah, 1999; Mowbray, Oyserman, Zemencuk, & Ross, 1995; Yonkers & Little, 2001).

Researchers and writers on psychological aspects of childbirth are rarely psychologists, and they generally do not identify psychologists as the type of practitioner best suited to help women prepare for or cope with the stressors of birthing. Instead, suggestions for clinical practice are usually intended for childbirth educators, nurses, midwives, or obstetricians so that they may identify problems and provide support, resources, and even counseling. Because there are many psychological aspects of birth, psychologists could play an important role in working to optimize women's experiences, through both research and clinical practice. Knowledge of current research about psychosocial aspects of childbirth will assist therapists in their efforts to help women prepare for, cope with, and process their childbirth experiences. This information should be helpful to practitioners who are working with women (a) who become pregnant during treatment, (b) for whom the pregnancy and birth have exacerbated or elucidated previous problems, and (c) who present with new difficulties as a result of a pregnancy and/or birth experience.

NORMATIVE ISSUES

Prenatal Anxiety

Researchers have investigated the effects of various forms or sources of anxiety, including state and trait anxiety and stressful life events, on women's health during pregnancy and on their birth outcomes. According to the authors of two thorough, critical literature reviews (Lobel, 1994; Paarlberg, Vingerhoets, Passchier, Dekker, & van Geijn, 1995), methodological flaws and inconsistencies make it difficult to draw solid conclusions regarding the impact of psychosocial stressors and anxiety during pregnancy on birth outcomes. However, stress and anxiety may be associated with numerous adverse outcomes such as preeclampsia, prolonged labor, preterm labor, and delivering a low birth weight infant. Hypothesized mediators of this complicated relationship include stress hormones, lifestyle behaviors such as smoking, and a suppressed immune system (Paarlberg et al., 1995).

What has been examined less frequently are anxieties specific to pregnancy and birth. Melender and Lauri (1999) interviewed Finnish women two to three days after they gave birth about their pregnancy and birth-related anxieties. Fears about pregnancy concerned fetal or infant health. Related to childbirth, women had been afraid of being alone and of experiencing pain and complications. Fearful reactions or emotions ranged from concern and uncertainty to terror, panic, and mild hysteria. Women also reported feeling depressed as a result of these fears. Healthy manifestations of fears included information seeking, whereas less healthy manifestations included crying and difficulty sleeping. In their study of 2,000 Swedish women who had either experienced a vaginal or a cesarean birth, Ryding, Wijma, Wijma, and Rydhstrom (1998) found that women who had cesarean sections scored significantly higher on measures of fears of childbirth and trait anxiety and lower on a measure of tolerance for stress. However, Crowe and von Baeyer (1989) actually found that women with high levels of fear both before and after a childbirth preparation series experienced less anxiety and pain during childbirth. A moderate level of anxiety during the last trimester of pregnancy may help women garner the coping resources they need and develop realistic expectations about labor and delivery.

Childbirth Experiences

Childbirth is a multidimensional life event, and women simultaneously report both negative and positive aspects of childbirth. These include pain, anxiety, and a loss of control, as well as a sense of accomplishment or mastery and enjoyment or satisfaction (Norr, Block, Charles, Meyering, & Meyers, 1977; Waldenstrom, Borg, Olsson, Skold, & Wall, 1996). As such, childbirth is regarded and described as a very powerful, important, memorable event (Johnston-Robledo & Donofrio, 1999; Peterson, 1996; Simkin, 1991). Typically, the stressors of giving birth do not extend beyond women's coping resources. Preparation for and social support during the birthing process are especially likely to facilitate coping and lead to positive outcomes such as perceived control, decreased pain and anxiety, and a more satisfying experience overall (Hart & Foster, 1997; Hillier & Slade, 1989; Johnston-Robledo, 1998; Lowe, 1989; Zhang, Bernasko, Leybovich, Fahs, & Hatch, 1996). Satisfaction with maternity care is another important component of a positive evaluation of the childbirth experience. Women tend to be more satisfied with their maternity care if it facilitates empowerment and an active role in decision making (Brown & Lumley, 1998; Green et al., 1990; Halldorsdottir & Karlsdottir, 1996; Seguin, Therrien, Champagne, & Larouche, 1989).

Regardless of whether their childbirth experiences are positive or negative, women are often eager to discuss them. DiMatteo, Kahn, and Berry (1993) provided postpartum women with an opportunity to discuss their birth experiences in focus groups. Themes of the discussions that the researchers identified included pain and emotional reactions that differed from what women expected; financial concerns; loss of autonomy and control; and the value of support during labor and birth. Fowles (1998) conducted interviews with women who were nine weeks postpartum about concerns they had regarding aspects of their labor and delivery experiences. Responses were categorized as different types of frustrations due to: pain, both from birthing and recovery; lack of control; lack of knowledge; and perceptions of negative interactions with health care providers. As a result of these interrelated concerns, some women expressed feelings of regret, anger, and overall dissatisfaction with their birth experiences.

Medical Interventions

Childbirth has become a medical and technological event, particularly in the United States, and, as a result, women may experience a variety of interventions. Minor interventions include shaving, enemas, fetal monitoring, intravenous antibiotics, and episiotomies. Major interventions include operative deliveries (forceps, vacuum extraction, cesarean), induction of labor, and anesthesia. Green et al. (1990) conducted a large prospective study on correlates of women's satisfaction with their childbirth experiences and their emotional well-being at six weeks postpartum. Obstetric interventions, both major and minor, were associated with less fulfilling, less satisfying experiences and a sense of feeling "out of control." The only intervention associated with decreased emotional well-being was a cesarean section. Contrary to popular belief, high expectations (e.g., utility of coping techniques, staying in control of self and events) were not associated with feelings of failure or disappointment.

Bramadat (1994) conducted an extensive literature review on women's experiences with and outcomes from induced labor (i.e., amniotomy and/or intravenous medication). She concluded that induced labor is often accompanied by other interventions such as anesthesia, operative deliveries, episiotomies, and fetal monitoring. Infants born after induced labor are more likely to experience problems such as jaundice and respiratory difficulties. Women describe induced labor as more painful than they expected and their birth experiences as worse than they expected. They may also be less likely to breastfeed their infants. Women who actually elect induced labor tend to have expectations of high anxiety during labor and an excessive need to feel safe.

The type of intervention that has received the most attention in the literature is a cesarean section, which, in the United States, accounts for approximately 24% of all deliveries (Nelson, 1996). In a meta-analysis of 43 empirical studies, DiMatteo et al. (1996) did not find a significant association between cesarean section and postpartum well-being. However, they concluded that such deliveries were associated with a variety of negative outcomes. These included decreased likelihood of breastfeeding, less fulfilling birth experience, less interaction with infant from one to five months postpartum, more fatigue up to two months postpartum, poorer physical functioning, and less maternal confidence at one month postpartum. The authors argued for the need to prepare women for the possibility of a cesarean section and its myriad psychosocial consequences.

Implications for Clinical Practice

The quality of women's experiences with childbirth may influence adjustment during the transition to parenthood (Mercer, 1986) and may have a long-term impact on their self-esteem and self-confidence (Simkin, 1991). Researchers are examining additional postpartum outcomes that may be influenced by women's birth experiences. In her review paper, Simkin (1996b) indicated that there is some evidence for postpartum mood, maternal-infant bonding, and breastfeeding to be negatively impacted by a dissatisfying birth experience.

Findings from these studies suggest the importance of encouraging women to discuss their goals, expectations, and plans for birth. Psychotherapists can also assist women in developing realistic expectations of the demands of childbirth and of their own performance during childbirth. Therapists can help women determine their personal meaning of birthing and which components of the birth are especially important to them. Assertiveness skills may help women communicate their needs during birth in order to avoid feeling out of control or uninvolved in important decisions. Therapists may encourage women to identify their needs and desires and communicate these to health care providers in the form of written birth plans. Springer (1996) found that women who wrote such a plan had slightly lower levels of state anxiety than women who did not. Therapists can help women cope during pregnancy by providing them with information about which emotional reactions are normal or to be expected and which may signal a need for intervention. Finally, women should be encouraged to process their birth experiences shortly after they occur. This opportunity may help them to reconcile ambivalent feelings about the experience, themselves, their partners, and their infants, and provide them with a chance to express any anger, violated expectations, or disappointments. Ambivalent feelings about birthing are likely, as many women experience unexpected events or sensations while giving birth. Even if psychotherapists do not play a direct role in the management of normative childbirth issues, they can certainly contribute to the development and evaluation of theory-based, empirically supported techniques for optimizing women's childbirth experiences. Wideman and Singer (1984) described the psychological principles utilized in traditional childbirth preparation such as conditioning, cognitive restructuring, and social support. They also speculated about additional psychological factors that may contribute to the efficacy of preparation such as social comparison, conformity, and perceived control. Wideman and Singer (1984) expressed their concerns about the lack of involvement of psychologists in the evaluation of these popular programs. Finally, social scientists should be more involved in researching women's birth experiences, which would ultimately inform both childbirth education and clinical practice.

CLINICAL ISSUES

Traumatic Birth Experiences

Researchers and practitioners are beginning to recognize that childbirth can be a traumatic event for some women (Ballard, Stanley, & Brockington, 1995; Creedy et al., 2000; Moleman, van der Hart, & van der Kolk, 1992; Radosti, 1999; Reynolds, 1997; Wijma et al., 1997). In her literature review, Radosti (1999) identified two types of trauma related to childbirth. In the first, or primary trauma, the birth experience itself is the traumatic event. She argued that the extremely personal nature of birthing, which can involve threats to a woman's physical safety, body image, and sexuality, and the intense emotions that accompany it render women vulnerable, particularly when they give birth in an impersonal setting. According to Radosti (1999) this context can lead to both emotional sources of trauma during birth (e.g., uncaring interactions with a health care provider, conflict with a spouse) and physical sources (e.g., threats to maternal or fetal health, surgery, and other interventions). The second type of trauma is retraumatization (Radosti, 1999). Women with a history of trauma experiences, particularly those related to a sexual trauma (e.g., childhood sexual abuse, sexual assault) are at risk of experiencing childbirth as traumatizing. The childbirth experience can either trigger or exacerbate symptoms from a previous traumatic event (Radosti, 1999).

Reactions to Traumatic Birth

A variety of reactions to a traumatic birth have been recognized; most of these have been described in relation to the primary trauma delineated by Radosti (1999). One of the earliest of these was the Partus Stress Reaction, identified by Moleman et al. (1992), which is similar to a brief reactive dissociative disorder. The authors reported three case studies in which women, all of whom had difficulty getting pregnant and complicated pregnancies, became extremely fearful of threats to their infants during childbirth. The panic was alleviated once the women entered a dissociative state. After birthing, these women continued to experience dissociation and amnesia in addition to nightmares, intrusive thoughts, and difficulty bonding with their infants.

A reaction more commonly reported is posttraumatic stress disorder (PTSD) (Ballard et al., 1995; Fones, 1996; Wijma et al., 1997). Prevalence rates of PTSD following birth are difficult to determine, as there are few large-scale studies reported in the literature. Ballard et al. (1995) reported four case studies in which women experienced PTSD as a result of birth experiences involving problems with the infant, problems with anesthesia, and excessive pain. In addition to the PTSD symptoms, all four women suffered from a depressive illness and/or other psychological problems such as hallucinations or pathological anxieties. In three of the cases, symptoms persisted for a year, and in two, women experienced difficulties interacting with their infants. Fones (1996) reported a case study of a woman who experienced PTSD symptoms for nine years after giving birth and developed a fear of subsequent childbirth that impacted her intimate relationship and her sexuality. In a large-scale study of over 1,600 Swedish women, Wijma et al. (1997) reported that 1.7% of the sample met the criteria for PTSD. This prevalence rate was determined using a scale of trauma specific to childbirth. The traumatized women were more likely to be first time mothers, to have received psychological counseling previously, and to have perceived negative interactions with medical staff during childbirth. In a qualitative study of British women's traumatic births, Allen (1998) found that 30% of her participants scored in the clinical range for reexperiencing and avoidance symptoms. She identified the loss of control as the primary reason why women perceive birth as traumatic. Extreme pain, fear of harm to self or baby, and past experiences all lead women to perceive a loss of control. Half of the sample had distress symptoms at 10 months postpartum. Reynolds (1997) also stated that extreme painfulness and loss of control, two features of many women's birth experiences, can lead to the experience of birthing as a traumatic event.

Creedy et al. (2000) found that 33% of a large sample of Swedish women reported some type of stressful or traumatic birthing event and three or more trauma symptoms. Six percent met the *DSM-IV* criteria for PTSD. Significant predictors of trauma symptoms included obstetrical interventions (e.g., emergency cesarean, forceps, vacuum extraction), dissatisfaction with the technical skill of health care providers, and dissatisfaction with partner support.

Childbirth as a Traumatic Event

Women who experience an emergency cesarean section are especially likely to report traumatic stress reactions (Ryding, Wijma, & Wijma, 1997, 1998a, 1998b). In their qualitative study of Swedish women's experiences, Ryding et al. (1997) found that 75% of participants perceived their emergency cesarean as traumatic both immediately afterward and two months postpartum. Fifty percent had experienced posttraumatic stress symptoms within the first two months postpartum, particularly those symptoms from the intrusion and arousal categories; but none of these women met *DSM-III* criteria for PTSD. Women who were most likely to perceive their caesareans as traumatic were those who reported having positive expectations that were violated and fears about birthing that were realized (Ryding, Wijma, & Wijma, 2000). As compared with the women who did not experience a posttraumatic stress reaction, those who did reported feeling "wronged" by the staff said they'd had a previous negative experience as a patient, and had a poor marital relationship (Ryding et al., 1998a). In a follow-up study (Ryding, Wijma, & Wijma, 1998c) with a larger sample, they found that 55% reported experiencing intense fear for their own or the baby's life. Other common reactions women had were feelings of "derealization" and disappointment. Twenty-six percent of the participants blamed themselves for the need to have a cesarean section.

Instrumental vaginal births, i.e., those that included forceps or vacuum extraction, have also been associated with traumatic stress reactions. Ryding et al. (1998b) found that women who had either an emergency cesarean section or experienced an instrumental vaginal birth reported more negative appraisals of the experience and higher levels of intrusive and avoidant symptoms at one month postpartum than women who had experienced a planned cesarean or a normal vaginal birth. Of those who underwent emergency caesareans, 5.6% scored in a clinical range for PTSD, as did 2.2% of the women who experienced an instrumental vaginal birth.

Given that an unplanned cesarean birth or instrumental vaginal birth can be very difficult if not traumatizing, would women prefer and request a planned cesarean section, particularly those women who have experienced a traumatic birth previously? From their critical literature review, Gamble and Creedy (2000) concluded that, unless women have experienced a previous complication, it is extremely unusual that they would request a cesarean. The authors question whether women really have control over their choices, as those who elect a cesarean may be influenced by the values of their health care provider.

In a study of 310 Australian women's preferences, Gamble and Creedy (2001) found that 6.4% of women preferred a cesarean, primarily on the basis of safety for the baby or a physician's recommendation. Almost all of these women either had a current complication or had experienced a complicated birth previously. These women also scored higher on state anxiety, were afraid of labor, and felt less prepared for birth. However, 68% of the women who had experienced a previous cesarean preferred a vaginal birth after a cesarean (VBAC).

Given that pregnancy and birth are associated with a happy, exciting time for women, they may be especially disappointed or even traumatized when complications arise and interventions are necessary. Starting from the very beginning, mothers are not supposed to focus on their own needs or complain. Therefore, new mothers may have a difficult time expressing their sense of disappointment or traumatic reactions to significant others. Sharing reactions to a bad experience may be especially difficult if significant others view complications and interventions during labor and delivery as "worth it" if a healthy baby is the result. Thus the potentially traumatizing effects of a birth experience on women may be unacknowledged or denied by others (Radosti, 1999). It is possible that this tendency to deny the significance of women's reactions to a traumatic birth may contribute to the dearth of empirical research on traumatic birth experiences.

A traumatic birth experience can impact women's postpartum functioning negatively. Allen's (1998) participants reported that the distress from their traumatic births led to feelings of panic, tearfulness, anger, and mistrust of others. The women in her study also noted that their relationships with their partners and infants were negatively affected by their distress. Almost half of her participants said they would not want more children because of their traumatic labor experiences. Reynolds (1997) noted that a traumatic birth had a negative impact on his clients' self-worth and impeded their ability to breastfeed, bond with their infants, and engage in sexual activity. Creedy et al. (2000) speculated about the possible effects of acute trauma symptoms on women's postpartum functioning. They argued that reexperiencing symptoms could impair women's adaptation to the maternal role, their relationships with other people, their ability to make decisions, and their general well-being. Avoidance symptoms can make it difficult for women to process their experiences and possibly lead to social isolation and an avoidance of helpful services. Finally, they postulated that arousal symptoms can lead to sleep disturbances, physical problems, and excessive concerns about the baby.

Retraumatization During Childbirth

Courtois and Riley (1992) argued that pregnancy and birth may serve as major triggers of childhood sexual abuse memories because of the psychological and physical characteristics of pregnancy and birth. In fact, Parratt (1994) noted that both CSA and childbirth involve intimate relationships, sexuality, and contact with the genitals. Furthermore, survivors of CSA may find that the vulnerable conditions of birth may be heightened. Aspects of birthing that CSA survivors may find particularly threatening include painful pelvic sensations, a lack of control, uncaring treatment by health care professionals, and exposure of their bodies (Radosti, 1999; Rhodes & Hutchinson, 1994; Seng & Hassinger, 1998). Any of these sensations or experiences can remind women, or lead to a reliving, of their abuse experiences. Simkin (1996a) noted that CSA survivors may experience discomfort with the manual examinations during labor and be apprehensive about breastfeeding their infants. They may also fear tearing during a vaginal delivery and, thus, prefer a cesarean.

In their study of health care providers' perceptions of birthing women who were CSA survivors, Rhodes and Hutchinson (1994) identified four different labor styles that these women tended to exhibit: fighting, taking control, surrendering, and retreating. They argued that these four styles represent extremes of the types of behaviors most laboring women who are not CSA survivors tend to exhibit. Others have indicated that some CSA survivors practice dissociation during labor and birth, which can actually lead to shorter labors (Parratt, 1994; VanDerLeden & Raskin, 1993). However, this technique may also prevent women from being active participants in the birth process and interfere with adjustment during the postpartum period (Cole, Scoville, & Flynn, 1996; Heritage, 1998).

The dearth of research on the impact of previous trauma on women's birth experiences makes it difficult if not impossible to make definitive statements about this complicated relationship. In one qualitative study of six women's experiences, Parratt (1994) found that the experience of childbirth did evoke abuse memories for these women, three of whom were unaware of the abuse until after birthing. She also found that certain aspects of the birth experience such as being touched during internal exams, lack of privacy, pain, and loss of control were likely either to evoke memories or to feel similar to a prior abuse experience. Jacobs (1992) compared the pregnancy experiences and birth outcomes of a small group of CSA survivors (n = 15) recruited from a mental health treatment program with those of a control group. He found that survivors were more likely to have had abortions, to have been younger when they first became pregnant, and to have experienced longer labors and more medical problems than the other women. Most important, the CSA survivors reported higher levels of perceived stress during pregnancy. This stress often arose from experiences with verbal, physical, and sexual abuse within a current interpersonal relationship.

Implications for Clinical Practice

Several authors (Creedy et al., 2000; Radosti, 1996; Reynolds, 1997) have made sound suggestions for helping women during pregnancy, birth, and postpartum who may be at risk for traumatic birth experiences. These suggestions were intended for health care professionals; however, we argue that psychotherapists are also in a position to contribute to women's mental health during this pivotal, vulnerable time in women's lives.

First, it is important that therapists obtain information during pregnancy about previous experiences that could contribute to a traumatic birth. These include previous reproductive difficulties such as a miscarriage or stillbirth, a history of sexual victimization, or an experience with PTSD (Radosti, 1999). In addition, realistic preparation for experiences and reactions women may have during childbirth may protect them from excessive concerns about feeling helpless or perceiving the impending birth as dangerous.

Given that women with previous traumatic birth experiences may elect a cesarean section (Gamble & Creedy, 2001; Ryding, 1993), psychotherapists can discuss the advantages and disadvantages of this option to help women make an informed choice or accept the fact that, because they are at risk, they may not have a choice. Reynolds (1997) argued that therapists may want to encourage women to attempt a normal vaginal birth, as a positive birth experience, or "redemptive birth" (p. 834), may be therapeutic. According to Gamble and Creedy (2000), women who are especially fearful of birth may need resources and encouragement from professionals, particularly from those who have a positive attitude toward normal birthing, that will help them prepare for and cope with a vaginal birth.

Therapists may help women at risk for a traumatic birth experience to manage pain and reinstate control during birthing by talking with them about their options and encouraging them to build trust with their health care providers. They may also want to help their clients seek obstetricians, midwives, and doulas, i.e., individuals trained to provide labor support, who are aware of and sensitive to the unique issues of women at risk for traumatic births.

During the postpartum period, psychotherapists can help women process their birth experiences in an attempt to determine whether they had a traumatic experience and to help them resolve any violated expectations. They should also assess for trauma symptoms so that a trauma syndrome can be identified and treated immediately. Therapists can also help reduce women's postbirth distress by encouraging coping strategies identified by Allen's (1998) participants as most helpful. These included reframing birthing events in a positive manner, making time for oneself, and accessing social support.

There are many ways that psychotherapists can support and guide CSA survivors during pregnancy, childbirth, and the postpartum period. Jacobs (1992) recommended that counselors prepare pregnant CSA survivors for the variety of fears, experiences, and complications that may occur as a result of their prior abuse experiences. For example, clients can be informed of the types of reactions to labor they may experience. They should also be informed of coping strategies, such as staying focused during labor and birthing, that may prevent the resurfacing of negative memories associated with pelvic or vaginal pain (Rhodes & Hutchinson, 1994). Psychotherapists can describe, as explicitly as possible, the pain and sensations that women may feel during labor and delivery so that women can anticipate what will happen and cope with these experiences. Clinicians can also help women with prior abuse histories to develop a birth plan that may help to reduce anxiety levels and create an environment within which they feel safe. Involvement in decisions about their births may minimize feelings of helplessness or loss of control (Heritage, 1998; Rhodes & Hutchinson, 1994). These plans may be derived from resources that CSA survivors (Parratt, 1994) and authors (Heritage, 1998; Rhodes & Hutchinson, 1994; Simkin, 1996a) have identified as helpful during birth. These can include privacy; continuity of care and a trusting relationship with a provider, possibly one who is not the same sex as the perpetrator; and special coping strategies for potentially uncomfortable procedures or phases of labor. It is also important that clinicians help CSA survivors prepare for how they will cope if their plans cannot be implemented during labor and birthing.

Therapists should also be aware of major mental health risks facing abuse survivors. According to Cole et al. (1996) these mental health risks include depression, dissociation, problems with infant attachment, and sexual dysfunction. Their recommendations for the well-being of pregnant CSA survivors, which are intended primarily for physical health care providers, are to screen pregnant women for current or previous abuse; assess for associated problems, both physical and psychological; provide psychotherapy to women, with particular attention paid to the aforementioned issues; and involve a team of health care providers. Psychotherapists, although not mentioned by the authors, are an essential component of such a team.

In order to validate women's experiences and assist them in the coping process, it is imperative that researchers conduct prospective studies to investigate the predictors of a traumatic birth, the impact of traumatic birth on women's adjustment, and unique issues of CSA survivors.

Psychotherapy During Pregnancy

Psychotherapists may play the most significant role in the psychological well-being of women with whom they are working during the course of the pregnancy. Women who may be especially in need of treatment during pregnancy include women with unplanned or untimely pregnancies; women who become pregnant as a result of a rape; women who have experienced prior obstetric difficulties such as a stillbirth; and women who are anticipating the birth of an unhealthy infant (Erlick & Wisner, 2001; Krueger, 1988; Raphael-Leff, 1990). Also at risk are women who have a poor quality intimate relationship, are victims of domestic violence, and are experiencing a large number of stressful life events (Gazmararian et al., 1996; Miller & Shah, 1999; Wilson et al., 1996). Psychotherapists working with pregnant clients should be mindful of these and other issues that place women at risk for adverse childbirth and postpartum outcomes; it is important to develop effective screening methods and interventions for these clients.

Women with a current psychological disorder or with a history of psychopathology also have unique needs during pregnancy. Pregnant women with major mental illnesses such as schizophrenia or depression are more likely to experience unplanned pregnancies, have inadequate emotional and tangible support, have a more difficult time accessing prenatal care, have poor nutrition, experience obstetric interventions, and have impaired postpartum psychological health and relationships with their infants (Miller & Shah, 1999; Mowbray et al., 1995). They will also have specific needs and concerns regarding the use of psychotropic medication during pregnancy and lactation (Altshuler & Szuba, 1994; Stewart & Erlick, 2001; Yolles, 2001). Women with eating disorders may be at higher risk than normal women for miscarriage, inappropriate weight gain, fetal and/or obstetric complications, excessive nausea and vomiting, and postpartum depression (Franko et al., 2001; Franko & Spurrell, 2000; Grady-Weliky, 2001). In addition, body weight and shape changes could disturb or depress women who were previously eating-disordered. Extensive coverage of psychopathologies among pregnant women is beyond the scope of this article. Stotland and Stewart (2001) and Yonkers and Little (2001) have edited books that cover a broad array of issues specific to psychiatric disorders and pregnancy.

CONCLUSION

There are many psychological aspects to pregnancy, birthing, and postpartum adjustment that psychotherapists have the background and skills necessary to address and investigate. The emphasis here on opportunities for psychotherapists to work with pregnant and postpartum women is by no means intended to imply that pregnancy, birth, and the postpartum period are crisis events that inevitably lead to psychological distress. However, these events potentially can render women vulnerable to a variety of adverse outcomes that affect their own mental health and that of their families in a profound way. Some women, such as those who are excessively anxious during pregnancy, women who experience a traumatic birth, childhood sexual abuse survivors, and women with underlying psychopathology, may be especially vulnerable to adverse outcomes. The psychological well-being of these childbearing women could be greatly enhanced by a treatment team that includes a therapist who is knowledgeable about and attentive to the plethora of unique psychological issues these women may face during pregnancy, birthing, and the postpartum period.

Although all women experience some degree of stress, challenge, and adjustment associated with pregnancy and childbirth and may benefit from working with a therapist, it may not be feasible for psychotherapists to become involved with women who experience a normal pregnancy and birth. However, psychotherapists can help optimize pregnancy and birth indirectly by the development and utilization of screening tools for depression or traumatic reactions related to birthing, as well as the development and evaluation of interventions, such as those intended to encourage breastfeeding, or facilitate adjustment to a challenging birth or during the postpartum period. They can also impart knowledge by volunteering as a guest speaker on psychological issues in a childbirth preparation series, providing in-service training to obstetric staff, and conducting support groups for women coping with a variety of childbearing issues.

REFERENCES

Allen, S. (1998). A qualitative analysis of the process, mediating variables, and impact of traumatic childbirth. *Journal of Reproductive and Infant Psychology, 16,* 107-131.

Altshuler, L. L., & Szuba, M. P. (1994). Course of psychiatric disorders in pregnancy: Dilemmas in pharmacologic management. *Neurological Clinics, 12,* 613-35.

Ballard, C. B., Stanley, A. K., & Brockington, I. F. (1995). Post-traumatic stress disorder (PTSD) after childbirth. *British Journal of Psychiatry, 166,* 525-528.

Bramadat, I. J. (1994). Induction of labor: An integrated review. *Health Care for Women International, 15,* 135-148.

Brown, S., & Lumley, J. (1998). Changing childbirth: Lessons from an Australian survey of 1336 women. *British Journal of Obstetrics and Gynecology, 105,* 143-155.

Cole, B. V., Scoville, M., & Flynn, L. T. (1996). Psychiatric advance practice nurses collaborate with certified nurse midwives in providing health care for pregnant women with histories of abuse. *Archives of Psychiatric Nursing, 10,* 229-234.

Courtois, C. A., & Riley, C. C. (1992). Pregnancy and childbirth as triggers for abuse memories: Implications for care. *Birth, 19,* 222-223.

Creedy, D. K., Shochet, I. M., & Horsfall, J. (2000). Childbirth and the development of acute trauma symptoms: Incidence and contributing factors. *Birth, 27,* 104-111.

Crowe, K., & von Baeyer, C. (1989). Predictors of a positive childbirth experience. *Birth, 16,* 59-63.

DiMatteo, M. R., Kahn, K. L., & Berry, S. H. (1993). Narratives of birth and the postpartum: Analysis of the focus group responses of new mothers. *Birth, 20,* 204-211.

DiMatteo, M. R., Morton, S. C., Lepper, H. S., Damush, T. M., Carney, M. F., Pearson, M. et al. (1996). Cesarean childbirth and psychosocial outcomes: A meta-analysis. *Health Psychology, 15,* 303-314.

Erlick, G. R., & Wisner, K. L. (2001). Fetal anomaly. In N. L. Stotland & D. E. Stewart (Eds.), *Psychological aspects of women's health care: The interface between psychiatry and obstetrics and gynecology* (2nd ed.) (pp. 33-50). Washington, DC: American Psychiatric Press.

Fones, C. (1996). Posttraumatic stress disorder occurring after painful childbirth. *Journal of Nervous and Mental Disease, 184,* 195-196.

Fowles, E. R. (1998). Labor concerns of women two months after delivery. *Birth, 25,* 235-240.

Franko, D. L., Blais, M. A., Becker, A. E., Delinsky, S. S., Greenwood, D. N., Flores, A. T. et al. (2001). Pregnancy complications and neonatal outcomes in women with eating disorders. *American Journal of Psychiatry, 158,* 1461-1466.

Franko, D. L., & Spurrell, E. B. (2000). Detection and management of eating disorders during pregnancy. *Obstetrics & Gynecology, 6,* 942-946.

Gamble, J. A., & Creedy, D. K. (2000). Women's request for a cesarean-section: A critique of the literature. *Birth, 27,* 256-263.

Gamble, J. A., & Creedy, D. K. (2001). Women's preference for a cesarean section: Incidence and associated factors. *Birth, 28,* 101-110.

Gazmararian, J. A., Lazorick, S., Spitz, A. M., Ballard, T. J., Saltzman, L.E., & Marks, J. A. (1996). Prevalence of violence against pregnant women. *Journal of the American Medical Association, 275,* 1915-1920.

Grady-Weliky, T. A. (2001). Eating disorders and hyperemesis gravidarum. In K. Yonkers & B. Little (Eds.), *Management of psychiatric disorders in pregnancy* (pp. 164-171). New York: Oxford University Press.

Green, J. M., Coupland, V. A., & Kitzinger, J. V. (1990). Expectations, experiences, and psychological outcomes of childbirth: A prospective study of 825 women. *Birth, 17,* 15-24.

Halldorsdottir, S., & Karlsdottir, S. I. (1996). Empowerment or discouragement: Women's experiences of caring and uncaring encounters during childbirth. *Health Care for Women International, 17,* 361-379.

Hart, M. A., & Foster, S. N. (1997). Couples' attitudes toward childbirth participation: Relationship to evaluation of labor and delivery. *Journal of Perinatal and Neonatal Nursing, 11,* 10-20.

Heritage, C. (1998). Working with childhood sexual abuse survivors during pregnancy, labor, and birth. *Journal of Obstetrics, Gynecology, and Neonatal Nursing, 27,* 671-677.

Hillier, C. A., & Slade, P. (1989). The impact of antenatal classes knowledge, anxiety, and confidence in primiparous women. *Journal of Reproductive and Infant Psychology, 7,* 3-13.

Jacobs, J. L. (1992). Child sexual abuse victimization and later sequelae during pregnancy and childbirth. *Journal of Child Sexual Abuse, 1,* 103-112.

Johnston-Robledo, I. (1998). Beyond Lamaze: Socioeconomic status and women's experiences with childbirth preparation. *Journal of Gender, Culture, and Health, 3,* 159-169.

Johnston-Robledo, I., & Donofrio, C. (1999, March). The role of socioeconomic status in women's birth stories. In H. Bullock (Chair), *Low income women: Connecting research, practice, and policy.* Symposium presented at the meeting of the Association for Women in Psychology, Providence, RI.

Krueger, M. M. (1988). Pregnancy as a result of rape. *Journal of Sex Education & Therapy, 14*, 23-27.

Lobel, M. (1994). Conceptualizations, measurement, and effects of prenatal maternal stress on birth outcomes. *Journal of Behavioral Medicine, 17*, 225-272.

Lowe, N. K. (1989). Explaining the pain of active labor: The importance of maternal confidence. *Research in Nursing and Health, 12*, 237-245.

Melender, H-L., & Lauri, S. (1999). Fears associated with pregnancy and childbirth-experiences of women who have recently given birth. *Midwifery, 15*, 177-182.

Mercer, R. T. (1986). *First-time motherhood experiences from teens to forties*. New York: Springer.

Miller, L. J. (2001). Psychiatric disorders during pregnancy. In N. L. Stotland & D. E. Stewart (Eds.), *Psychological aspects of women's health care: The interface between psychiatry and obstetrics and gynecology* (2nd ed.) (pp. 51-66). Washington, DC: American Psychiatric Press.

Miller, L. J., & Shah, A. (1999). Major mental illness during pregnancy. *Primary Care Update for Ob/Gyns, 6*, 163-168.

Moleman, N., van der Hart, O., & van der Kolk, B. A. (1992). The partus stress reaction: A neglected etiological factor in postpartum psychiatric disorders. *Journal of Nervous and Mental Disease, 180*, 271-272.

Mowbray, C. T., Oyserman, D., Zemencuk, J. K., & Ross, S. R. (1995). Motherhood for women with serious mental illness: Pregnancy, childbirth, and the postpartum period. *American Journal of Orthopsychiatry, 65*, 21-38.

Nelson, E. J. (1996). The American experience of childbirth. In R. L. Parrott & C. M. Condit (Eds.), *Evaluating women's health messages* (pp. 109-123). Thousand Oaks, CA: Sage.

Norr, K. L., Block, C. R., Charles, A., Meyering, S., & Meyers, E. (1977). Explaining pain and enjoyment in childbirth. *Journal of Health and Social Behavior, 18*, 260-275.

Paarlberg, K. M., Vingerhoets, J. J. M., Passchier, J., Dekker, G. A., & van Geijn, H. P. (1995). Psychosocial factors and pregnancy outcome: A review with emphasis on methodological issues. *Journal of Psychosomatic Research, 39*, 563-595.

Parratt, J. (1994). The experience of childbirth for survivors of incest. *Midwifery, 10*, 26-39.

Peterson, G. (1996). Childbirth-The ordinary miracle: Effects of devaluation of childbirth on women's self-esteem and family relationships. *Pre- and Perinatal Psychology Journal, 11*, 101-109.

Radosti, S. (1999, April 30). The dynamics of trauma in childbirth. *Special Delivery, 22*, 2-7.

Raphael-Leff, J. (1990). Psychotherapy and pregnancy. *Journal of Reproductive and Infant Psychology, 8*, 119-135.

Reynolds, J. L. (1997). Post-traumatic stress disorder after childbirth: The phenomenon of traumatic birth. *Canadian Medical Association Journal, 156*, 831-835.

Rhodes, N., & Hutchinson, S. (1994). Labor experiences of childhood sexual abuse survivors. *Birth, 21,* 213-220.

Ryding, E. L. (1993). Investigation of 33 women who demanded a cesarean section for personal reasons. *Acta Obstetricia Gynecologica Scandinavica, 72,* 280-285.

Ryding, E. L., Wijma, B., & Wijma, K. (1997). Posttraumatic stress reactions after emergency cesarean section. *Acta Obstetricia Gynecologica Scandinavica, 76,* 856-861.

Ryding, E. L., Wijma, K., & Wijma, B. (1998a). Predisposing psychological factors for posttraumatic stress reactions after emergency cesarean section. *Acta Obstetricia Gynecologica Scandinavica, 77,* 351-352.

Ryding, E. L., Wijma, K., & Wijma, B. (1998b). Psychological impact of emergency cesarean section in comparison with elective cesarean section, instrumental, and normal vaginal delivery. *Journal of Psychosomatic Obstetrics and Gynecology, 19,* 135-144.

Ryding, E. L., Wijma, K., & Wijma, B. (1998c). Experiences of emergency cesarean section: A phenomenological study of 53 women. *Birth, 25,* 246-251.

Ryding, E. L., Wijma, K., & Wijma, B. (2000). Emergency cesarean section: 25 women's experiences. *Journal of Reproductive and Infant Psychology, 18,* 33-39.

Ryding, E. L., Wijma, B., Wijma, K., & Rydhstrom, H. (1998). Fear of childbirth during pregnancy may increase the risk of emergency cesarean section. *Acta Obstetricia Gynecologica Scandinavica, 77,* 542-547.

Seguin, L., Therrien, R., Champagne, F., & Larouche, D. (1989). The components of women's satisfaction with maternity care. *Birth, 16,* 109-113.

Seng, J. S., & Hassinger, J. A. (1998). Relationship strategies and interdisciplinary collaboration: Improving maternity care with survivors of childhood sexual abuse. *Journal of Nurse-Midwifery, 43,* 287-295.

Simkin, P. (1991). Just another day in a woman's life? Women's long-term perceptions of their first birth experience. *Birth, 18,* 203-210.

Simkin, P. (1996a). Childbirth education and care for the childhood sexual abuse survivor. *International Journal of Childbirth Education, 11,* 31-33.

Simkin, P. (1996b). The experience of maternity in a woman's life. *Journal of Obstetrics, Gynecology, and Neonatal Nursing, 25,* 247-252.

Springer, D. (1996). Birth plans: The effect on anxiety in pregnant women. *International Journal of Childbirth Education, 11,* 20-25.

Stewart, D. E., & Erlick, G. R. (2001). Psychotropic drugs and electroconvulsive therapy during pregnancy and lactation. In N. L. Stotland & D. E. Stewart (Eds.), *Psychological aspects of women's health care: The interface between psychiatry and obstetrics and gynecology* (2nd ed.) (pp. 67-93). Washington, DC: American Psychiatric Press.

Stotland, N. L., & Stewart, D. E. (Eds.). (2001). *Psychological aspects of women's health care: The interface between psychiatry and obstetrics and gynecology* (2nd ed.). Washington, DC: American Psychiatric Press.

VanDerLeden, M., & Raskin, V. (1993). Psychological sequelae of childhood abuse: Relevant in subsequent pregnancy. *American Journal of Obstetrics and Gynecology, 168,* 1336-1337.

Waldenstrom, U., Borg, I., Olsson, B., Skold, M., & Wall, S. (1996). The childbirth experience: A study of 295 new mothers. *Birth, 23*, 144-153.

Wideman, M. V., & Singer, J. E. (1984). The role of psychological mechanisms in preparation for childbirth. *American Psychologists, 39*, 1357-1371.

Wijma, K., Soderquist, M. A., & Wijma, B. (1997). Posttraumatic stress disorder after childbirth: A cross sectional study. *Journal of Anxiety Disorders, 11*, 587-597.

Wilson, L. M., Reid, A. J., Midmer, D. K., Biringer, A., Carroll, J. C., & Stewart, D. E. (1996). Antenatal psychosocial risk factors associated with adverse postpartum family outcomes. *Canadian Medical Association Journal, 154*, 785-799.

Yolles, J. C. (2001). Psychotropics versus psychotherapy: An individualized treatment plan for the pregnant patient. In K. Yonkers & B. Little (Eds.), *Management of psychiatric disorders in pregnancy* (pp. 1-16). New York: Oxford University Press.

Yonkers, K., & Little, B. (Eds.). (2001). *Management of psychiatric disorders in pregnancy*. New York: Oxford University Press.

Zhang, J., Bernasko, J. W., Leybovich, E., Fahs, M., & Hatch, M. C. (1996). Continuous labor support from labor attendant for primiparous women: A meta-analysis. *Obstetrics & Gynecology, 88*, 739-744.

Myths and Mates
in Childbearing Depression

Valerie E. Whiffen

SUMMARY. Many myths exist about postpartum depression (PPD), all of which are based on the assumption that PPD differs qualitatively from depression that occurs at other times in women's lives. These myths paint a misleading picture of how PPD arises and may prevent women from receiving treatment for their difficulties. In this article, I identify five common myths and review the research literature to demonstrate that each lacks an empirical basis. Next, I present a model based on attachment theory, which I use to conceptualize PPD that occurs in the context of relationship distress. Finally, I illustrate this model with a clinical case. *[Article copies available for a fee from The Haworth Document Delivery Service: 1-800-HAWORTH. E-mail address: <docdelivery@haworthpress.com> Website: <http://www.HaworthPress. com> © 2004 by The Haworth Press, Inc. All rights reserved.]*

KEYWORDS. Postpartum depression, attachment, marital distress

Valerie E. Whiffen, PhD, is Professor in the School of Psychology and Director of the APA-accredited Training Clinic at the University of Ottawa. She has published widely in the area of depression, with a particular focus on the causes of women's depression. She is a registered clinical psychologist, and has a small private practice for the treatment of depression and marital distress.

Address correspondence to: Valerie E. Whiffen, School of Psychology, University of Ottawa, Ottawa, ON K1N 6N5, Canada (E-mail: whiff@uottawa.ca).

[Haworth co-indexing entry note]: "Myths and Mates in Childbearing Depression." Whiffen, Valerie E. Co-published simultaneously in *Women & Therapy* (The Haworth Press, Inc.) Vol. 27, No. 3/4, 2004, pp. 151-164; and: *From Menarche to Menopause: The Female Body in Feminist Therapy* (ed: Joan C. Chrisler) The Haworth Press, Inc., 2004, pp. 151-164. Single or multiple copies of this article are available for a fee from The Haworth Document Delivery Service [1-800-HAWORTH, 9:00 a.m. - 5:00 p.m. (EST). E-mail address: docdelivery@haworthpress.com].

http://www.haworthpress.com/store/product.asp?sku=J015
10.1300/J015v27n03_11

151

> *What the laws of Texas have failed to realize is that pregnancy and birth*
> *involve one of the most massive physiological change[s] a human can*
> *experience. Motherhood is unique given the incredible flux of reproduc-*
> *tive hormones related to birth and the postpartum period. For some,*
> *these hormones lead to severe depression and psychosis. To say*
> *"Andrea Yates is sick and dangerous" simply ignores the existence of*
> *these reproductive flows which can bring feelings of great warmth and*
> *love in some, but also oppressive irrational thoughts and acts in others.*
> (Press release issued by Postpartum Support International, March 15,
> 2002)

The Andrea Yates case catapulted postpartum depression (PPD) onto the front pages of North American newspapers. It happens every time a young mother murders her infant. Often, as is true in this case, the children do not need even to be infants for the mother's behavior to be explained by PPD. The press release quoted above makes reference to many of the myths about depression that is related to childbirth. One of the primary myths adopted by medical professionals and promulgated by the media is that PPD is caused by biological factors, particularly hormones (Martinez, Johnston-Robledo, Ulsh, & Chrisler, 2000), a myth that persists despite the lack of evidence for a direct link. Collectively these myths create a picture of PPD that is at best misleading and at worst an impediment to effective treatment. However, medical professionals and the media are not the only ones who subscribe to these myths; their power is such that women with PPD often believe the myths themselves.

The myths all assume that PPD is different from nonchildbearing depression. However, a review of the research literature indicates that PPD has not been differentiated from depression that occurs at other points in women's lives. Similar to other episodes of depression, PPD often is associated with relationship difficulties.[1] In the second part of this article, I present a model of PPD that occurs in the context of relationship distress, which I illustrate with an example from my clinical work. Throughout the article, I highlight the implications of research and theory for psychotherapists who work with PPD women.

THE MYTHS OF POSTPARTUM DEPRESSION

Myth #1: Recently Delivered Women Are at Risk for PPD

The press release says it bluntly: Hormones associated with pregnancy and delivery cause childbearing women to be uniquely susceptible to depression. In popular press articles, hormones are cited more frequently than any other potential cause (Martinez et al., 2000). What is the empirical support for this assertion? Despite the persistence of hormonal explanations in the medical and lay literatures, there is surprisingly little evidence to support the role of hormones in the etiology of CBD. Some women experience CBD as a result of thyroid problems (Harris et al., 1989). However, no other hormonal causes have been identified consistently, despite decades of research on this topic.

Women are more prone to depression during childbearing periods than at other times in their lives. Approximately 13% of women who recently gave birth experience depressive symptoms severe enough to warrant a diagnosis of depression, which is a significant increase over the rate normally found among women of childbearing age (cf. Whiffen, 1992). However, to make sense of this number we need to distinguish *prevalence* from *incidence*. Prevalence rates refer to the total number of cases identified in the postpartum period regardless of when the episodes started, whereas incidence rates refer only to those cases that began after delivery. This distinction is critical because the label "postpartum depression" implies that the depression started after the partum event. However, studies that follow women from pregnancy show that as many as 40% of the episodes that are present after the birth *also were present during the pregnancy* (Whiffen, 1992). Researchers rarely make this distinction or attempt to date the onset of the episode. Thus, a depressive episode that is detected after childbirth could have begun at any time before, during, or after pregnancy, and therefore may or may not be related to having a baby.

The term "postpartum depression" is misleading because it implies that the depression is related causally to having a baby. This mislabeling can lead clinicians to misunderstand the nature of their client's depressive episodes. In recognition of this problem, I prefer the more descriptive term "childbearing depression" (CBD), which makes no assumptions about when the episode started. Using this term also reminds me as a clinician that, in trying to understand a childbearing woman's depression, I need to take into account not only her entire pregnancy but also the context in which she became pregnant. I am careful to investigate the possibility that the pregnancy is irrelevant to the depression.

Myth #2:
PPD Is Qualitatively Different from Other Forms of Depression

Some people argue that the symptoms of PPD are different from those of depression that occurs at other times, that women with PPD are more anxious and agitated, that they are obsessed with thoughts of harming their babies, or that they are at risk for infanticide. The specific connection between PPD and infanticide is made frequently in the popular press (Martinez et al., 2000). Groups that promote the study and treatment of PPD believe that they are more likely to get funding if they can make the case that PPD is a disorder to which childbearing women are uniquely susceptible. Admitting that PPD is not special may leave these women untreated, as are most women who experience depression (Hunsley, Lee, & Aubry, 1999). Although it is vital to obtain services for women with PPD, the argument that PPD is a unique disorder is a double-edged sword because it fosters the perception, widely held among medical professionals and in the media, that PPD is hormonal and self-correcting.

Is PPD different from other forms of depression? It is interesting that when CBD and depressed but nonchildbearing women are compared, there are few differences (Whiffen & Gotlib, 1993). CBD women tend to be less severely depressed than nonchildbearing depressed women, with an average score on the Beck Depression Inventory in the mild to moderate range. Less than half of the depressed women diagnosed in research studies meet criteria for Major Depression; the majority meet criteria for an Adjustment Disorder with Depressed Mood or Minor Depression. However, the types of symptoms they report, the courses of their episodes, and their scores on such psychosocial variables as coping and social support are indistinguishable from those of nonchildbearing depressed women. Thus, CBD typically is mild but does not seem to differ qualitatively from depression that occurs at other times, at least on the variables assessed by researchers to date. The major implication of this finding is that working with CBD women should be no different from working with women who are depressed at other times in their lives. Effective treatments for depression also should be effective for CBD, and the underlying causes of the depression should be basically the same.

Myth #3: PPD Does Not Need to Be Treated

Many medical professionals agree with the assertion that hormones cause CBD. Furthermore, they believe that women's mood will self-correct as their hormones return to pre-pregnancy levels. This perception may be part of the reason that most women do not receive treatment for CBD (Cox, Connor, & Kendell, 1982), although it is not clear that childbearing depressed women are any less likely to receive treatment than are nonchildbearing depressed women. However, in the absence of a hormonal explanation for CBD, there is no reason to believe that episodes remit spontaneously. Half of the episodes detected at 1 month postpartum are still present 5 months later, a recovery rate that does not differ from that for depressed but nonchildbearing women (Whiffen & Gotlib, 1993).

Perhaps CBD doesn't need to be treated because it is typically mild? Although the symptoms are mild, CBD is not a trivial disorder. Women who experience CBD are at risk for subsequent depressive episodes, both after pregnancy and at other times in their lives (Bagedahl-Strindlund & Ruppert, 1998). Between one-quarter and one-half of the women who experience an episode of CBD will have a depressive episode after a subsequent pregnancy (Cooper & Murray, 1995; Marks, Wieck, Checkley, & Kumar, 1996; Wisner et al., 2001). The median age of onset for a first episode of depression is 26 years (Burke, Burke, Regier, & Rae, 1990), which is close to the average age of 28 at which women in Western societies have their first children. Thus,

CBD may be the first episode of depression in the life of a woman who is vulnerable. This makes it an important episode to treat because the risk of relapse increases with each episode experienced (Teasdale et al., 2000).

An episode of depression at this point in a woman's life also can have enduring consequences for the infant and for the vitality of the woman's relationship with her partner. The infants of CBD women develop more slowly, and they cry more and are more difficult to soothe than the infants of nondepressed women (Beck, 1998; Whiffen & Gotlib, 1989b). It is not surprising that they also are less likely to form secure attachments to their mothers (Atkinson et al., 2000). Developmental psychologists believe that attachment security is a cornerstone of social and emotional adjustment in childhood. Thus, the infants of CBD women are at risk for emotional difficulties themselves. Finally, women who experience CBD continue to report lower levels of marital satisfaction 5 years later (Nettelbladt, Uddenberg, & Englesson, 1985). Thus, an episode of CBD can be associated with serious and long-lasting consequences for the woman as well as her family. Although the depressive symptoms may appear to be mild, because of its timing CBD often has a cascading impact on women's lives.

Myth #4:
PPD Occurs Suddenly to Otherwise Emotionally Healthy Women

Some writers describe CBD as a disorder that descends mysteriously and unpredictably from the heavens, a view that often is shared by the women who experience it. This impression simply is not supported by research. The best predictors of a new episode of PPD are a history of emotional problems and depression levels during pregnancy (O'Hara & Swain, 1996; Whiffen, 1992). The majority of women who develop CBD have sought help for emotional problems in the past, and they report higher levels of emotional distress during pregnancy than do women who do not develop CBD. Women also are more likely to become depressed when they experience during the childbearing period significant life stress that may or may not be related to pregnancy and/or to infant care (cf. Swendsen & Mazure, 2000). These are the same factors that are implicated in the onset of nonchildbearing depression (O'Hara, Schlechte, Lewis, & Varner, 1991), which lends further support to the lack of a distinction between CBD and other forms of depression.

The interpersonal context in which a woman lives also is a significant determinant of whether or not she will develop CBD. Women are more vulnerable if they believe that their childhood relationships with their parents lacked warmth or were explicitly rejecting (Gotlib, Whiffen, Wallace, & Mount, 1991). Among children, parental rejection is associated with the development of insecure attachment (Ainsworth, Blehar, Waters, & Wall, 1968), which may be a risk factor for adult depression (Whiffen, Kallos-Lilly, & MacDonald, 2001). Lack of social support, particularly lack of concrete help provided by the baby's father, also contributes to CBD (O'Hara & Swain, 1996). Lack of support may be an expression of marital distress, which is another reliable predictor of CBD (O'Hara & Swain, 1996; Whiffen, 1992). In one study, the husbands of women who went on to experience CBD were rated by interviewers during pregnancy as showing greater *indifference* toward their wives (Marks et al., 1996). They were not more critical or hostile, but they were more detached and less invested in their wives' pregnancies. Research with nonchildbearing depressed women indicates that husbands' indifference maintains or exacerbates wives' depression over time (Whiffen et al., 2001). In my clinical experience, women perceive husbands who are emotionally detached and unwilling to help with the care of a new baby as unloving. This attribution may be particularly painful if the woman believes that her parents rejected her as well.

Myth #5: Only Women Experience PPD

The implication that depression follows from a "partum" event, as well as the tendency to consider PPD a unique or hormonal disorder, leads most researchers to overlook the data that show that fathers of new babies also experience emotional distress. Men do not have a "partum" event, so they cannot develop PPD per se. Nonclinical studies show that having a baby is measurably more disruptive for fathers than it is for mothers. Although mothers' scores on measures of emotional distress and marital dissatisfaction return to their prepartum levels by one year postpartum, fathers' scores continue to indicate distress (Vandell, Hyde, Plant, & Essex, 1997). Three to nine percent of new fathers meet diagnostic criteria for an Axis I disorder, especially depression or anxiety (Ballard, Davis, Cullen, Mohan, & Dean, 1994), which is much higher than the usual rate for men of this age (e.g., Regier et al., 1988). In one sample of men whose wives already were diagnosed with depression, 1 in 4 of the husbands also met criteria for an Axis I disorder (Zelkowitz & Milet, 1996).

These findings are important even to a clinician who works exclusively with women because most childbearing women have an ongoing relationship with their baby's father. A depressed or anxious husband is likely to have a negative impact on his wife. When husbands are depressed, they tend to feel unhappy in their marriages. Husbands' marital distress tends to make their wives unhappy as well (Thompson, Whiffen, & Blain, 1995; Whiffen & Gotlib, 1989a), and a woman's marital dissatisfaction is a strong predictor of her subsequent experience of an episode of major depression (Whisman, 1999). In addition, the high rate of paternal diagnosis when mothers are depressed suggests that maternal depression may be a marker of a distressed *system*. Thus, it is important to consider the system that provides the immediate context for childbearing depression when treating these women.

WHAT IS CHILDBEARING DEPRESSION?

If CBD is not what the myths say it is, then what is it? So far, I have used the research to counteract the picture of CBD that is widely endorsed by medical professionals and promoted by the media (Martinez et al., 2000). Can we read between the lines of these studies to get a picture of what CBD is? Before doing so, it is important to emphasize that CBD is just as heterogeneous as depression that occurs at other times. One woman became depressed because her father developed terminal cancer shortly after she became pregnant. She passed her pregnancy worrying that he would die before she could give birth to her baby, his first grandchild. When he died 2 months after the birth, she plunged into a deep bereavement. Another woman became depressed when she had a little girl. Her first baby was a boy, and she experienced no depression related to that pregnancy. When her little girl was born she was reminded of the sexual abuse that she had experienced throughout her childhood. She grieved for her daughter's vulnerability to sexual victimization, and for her own abuse, which she had never processed. These vignettes show that there are as many causes of CBD as there are causes of nonchildbearing depression.

That having been said, the research does suggest certain patterns. The typical woman who experiences CBD is emotionally vulnerable. She feels rejected by one or both parents. She is unhappy in her romantic relationship and may fear that her partner does not really love her. She feels unsupported by her partner. Perhaps her partner does not help out around the house or with taking care of other children. Outsiders may see her partner as indifferent to her, and this indifference is likely to maintain her feelings of depression. These factors would (and do) induce depression at any point in a woman's life. Feminist theories maintain that women's self-concept and self-esteem are embedded in the context of their significant relationships (Miller, 1986). When women are able to maintain close and harmonious relationships with the people who are important to them, they feel good about themselves. Conversely, relationships that are disconnected or conflicted promote the development of low self-esteem and depression (Jack, 1991). I maintain that this process is heightened during childbearing periods. Pregnancy makes a woman especially vulnerable to relationship distress because the baby is a tangible manifestation of her commitment to her partner, and she will be sensitive to any indication that this commitment is not shared.

Attachment theory provides an interpersonal framework for conceptualizing and treating CBD when it occurs in the context of relationship distress (Whiffen & Johnson, 1998). Attachment theory developed originally as a description of infant-caregiver relationships. In the past 15 years, it has been extended to the study of romantic relationships, and it is now being applied to the treatment of clinical problems in couples and families (cf. Johnson & Whiffen, in press). Attachment theory proposes that both one's sense of self and one's beliefs about the availability and emotional responsiveness of others are determined by the quality of key relationships (Bowlby, 1969, 1973). As children we learn that we are lovable and that others are reliable and responsive to our needs by having parents or other attachment figures who treat us warmly and who demonstrate interest in and concern for us. Needs to feel connected to and accepted by significant others are not manifestations of dependency but basic human needs that are present throughout the lifespan. In Western societies where nuclear families predominate, the romantic partner is the primary attachment figure for most adults (Bartholomew, 1990; Hazan & Shaver, 1987). Partners who are warm and emotionally available mirror an image of ourselves as lovable and worthy, whereas those who are cold, critical, and disengaged reflect back a picture of ourselves as unlovable, defective, and unworthy. When our interactions with attachment figures tell us that we are unlovable or unimportant, we become distressed. We still attempt to meet our needs for connection and validation in our close relationships. However, when these relationships are distressed, our attempts may take maladaptive forms that inadvertently maintain or exacerbate emotional distress.

Attachment needs become particularly salient during transitions, which bring uncertainty and change and which prompt us to turn to attachment figures for reassurance (Bowlby, 1973). The introduction of a new child into an existing couple or family is a transition that can have dramatic consequences for couples' attachment security (Whiffen & Johnson, 1998). The birth of the first child has special implications for attachment because couples must relinquish their exclusive pair bond to become a family. First time mothers also want to feel good about their mothering, and they typically look to their partners for feedback about how well they are doing. A critical or unsupportive partner can undermine women's developing self-efficacy in the maternal role. Thus, for first time parents, the birth of a child has an impact both on their relationship and on the woman's sense of self. However, even couples with other children may find that the addition of a new baby creates emotional distance or challenges the mother's ability to cope. The way that a couple handles the birth of their children is an important test of their ability to remain emotionally available and responsive to one another under stressful conditions.

When individuals are stressed, they normally turn to an attachment figure for reassurance and comfort. According to the theory, this is one of the primary purposes served by attachment figures. In stressful circumstances, couples that are securely attached turn to one another and provide the reassurance that each person is seeking (cf. Johnson & Whiffen, 1999). Although securely attached couples may encounter difficulties associated with childbearing, they should be able to use their relationship to cope with stress and to regulate the associated negative affect. Thus, partners who have proven to one another in the past that they are emotionally available and responsive during periods of crisis should be relatively resilient to CBD. However, couples that have failed previous tests of their emotional availability will encounter difficulties. These failed tests may be "attachment injuries" (Johnson, Makinen, & Millikin, 2001) from a previous time in the relationship that have never been resolved. The birth of a new child also may trigger attachment fears in an individual who experienced disappointment and unavailability earlier in life with other figures. For instance, a woman who believes that her parents left her to fend for herself as a child may expect her partner to do the same.

Attachment insecurity takes one of two basic forms. Individuals who are *anxiously* attached to their romantic partners look to them frequently for reassurance because they believe they are unlovable. They are thought to have experienced inconsistency with attachment figures previously, which has left them vigilant to signs that they might be abandoned. Paradoxically, research shows that they tend to seek reassurance by blaming and criticizing their partners, in part because they have difficulty containing their high levels of negative emotion (cf. Johnson & Whiffen, 1999). This interpersonal coping strategy increases relationship conflict, which is strongly predictive of subsequent depression (Whisman, 1999).

Individuals who are *fearfully* attached to their romantic partners want to be close but fear that they will be rejected, a dilemma that they resolve by maintaining emotional distance even in their close relationships. When stressed, they tend to withdraw emotionally and physically from their partners (cf. Johnson & Whiffen, 1999). This interpersonal coping strategy may indicate that the individual is already on the road to depression; Bowlby (1980) considered giving up on the attachment figure to be the first step in the development of depression. This strategy also may create a self-fulfilling prophesy. Partners may not recognize fearfully attached individuals' distress and therefore neglect to provide the needed support. Partners' failure to provide support will confirm fearful individuals' perception that partners are unresponsive. This perception is likely to contribute to feelings of depression. Research with nonchildbearing couples indicates that fearful attachment is especially associated with depression when a fearful woman has a dismissing romantic partner or spouse (Whiffen et al., 2001). *Dismissing* individuals are thought to protect their self-esteem from the damaging effects of rejection by denying that attachment needs are important. Dismissing husbands are likely to be unaware of wives' distress and need for support and to respond insensitively to those bids for reassurance that they do recognize.

Depression is the most common form of emotional distress that women experience during childbearing periods. Bowlby (1980) linked sadness and depression specifically to loss and disappointment. The potential for loss and disappointment during childbearing periods is substantial despite cultural pressure to view the birth of a child as a joyful event that marks the beginning of a new life (Nicolson, 1998). Although the event is a beginning for the infant, it may be an ending for the parents. The transition from romantic couple to working partnership may be unexpected or come too early in the relationship for first time parents. The mother may stop working outside the home and have to give up not only the work role but also the social support and self-efficacy that work provides. Even a woman who previously stayed at home with small children may feel her life is suddenly constrained by a baby who has medical problems or who cries frequently. Change always is accompanied to some degree by loss. It is important for therapists to keep the idea of loss in mind when working with childbearing women because clients may believe that they are not entitled to experience and express feelings of loss about the beginning of their child's life.

Clinical Case

Annie was a professional woman in her 30s who had been married for about 18 months when she became pregnant. Her husband, Rob, was a U.S. citizen who had been unable to obtain a work permit in Canada, with the result that he had been unemployed for more than a year when I first saw her.

She was the third child in a family of five. Her mother was a stay-at-home mom who developed a terminal illness and died when Annie was an adolescent. Her father was a workaholic who was harshly critical of his children. Annie reported a weak attachment to her mother whom she perceived as overwhelmed by looking after her children. Even as a child, Annie was quick to withdraw from relationships if she felt hurt, angry, or disappointed. As an adult, she felt distant in her relationships with men. She said that she cultivated this distance, both because she found men's emotional demands overwhelming and because she was afraid of being hurt. Being married to Rob was a relief at first because he demanded very little emotional intimacy. In attachment terms, Annie reported a fearful style, and she described Rob as dismissing.

When Annie was approximately 7 months pregnant, she and Rob went on a canoeing trip with several other couples. On the second day, Annie fell and broke her wrist. Rob took her back to the base lodge, got her medical attention, bought her some novels, then announced that he was finishing the trip and would return in 5 days. Annie was devastated. This trip became an attachment injury to which Annie returned repeatedly during therapy. She believed that Rob's behavior reflected his lack of investment in her pregnancy. The incident had an extra emotional kick for her because the basis of their relationship was doing physical activities together. There was little emotional intimacy, and they had few common intellectual interests; Annie feared that without the glue of shared outdoor activities he would eventually find someone who was "more fun to play with." Through our work on this incident, Annie realized that she wanted to feel like a family with Rob instead of feeling like "separate checks."

When the baby was born, Annie's belief that he was not invested in her or the baby intensified because she saw him "carrying on with his life as if nothing (has) changed." She believed that she and the baby were unimportant to Rob and that eventually he would leave them both. She was aware of "shoring up her defenses" in preparation for this loss. For instance, she would not let him help in any way with the care of their child. She told me that she was afraid that if she put down part of her burden and let him pick it up, it would be too heavy to pick up again when he finally left her. By this time she was severely depressed.

In couples therapy we explored how Rob felt about becoming a father, and his behavior was immediately comprehensible: He was angry with Annie for getting pregnant. He thought that they had not been married long enough, and he wanted to be employed before becoming a father. They had one conversation about getting pregnant during which he expressed his feelings clearly, but Annie decided that he would change his mind once he became a father, and she stopped using birth control without telling him. Once she was pregnant, Rob thought that there was no point to repeatedly expressing his anger and disappointment. However, he could not embrace a decision that he had not made.

Rob's and Annie's attachment styles were compatible as long as they could lead relatively independent lives. Once they needed to become interdependent, neither believed that the other could be counted upon to be emotionally available and responsive. Annie felt unsupported and deserted by Rob, even though she reported that his behavior did not change much before and after the baby's birth. In fact, it was the lack of change when change was normative and expected that led her to believe that he was not invested in her pregnancy and their child. In Bowlby's terms, Annie's depression was linked to her loss of Rob when he failed to make the transition to parent with her. Rob thought that he had been treated as a "sperm bank." He also lost Annie in that she completely disregarded what he wanted, which led him to question how much she really cared for him as a person and how much he was just a "bit player" in her life.

CONCLUSION

The myths of PPD are all premised on the assumption that PPD is unique and different from nonchildbearing depression. However, a review of the research literature indicates that it is just like depression that occurs at other times in women's lives. Like nonchildbearing depression, the causes of CBD are varied, but a significant proportion of CBD women experience relationship difficulties. Relationship distress is depressing because most women's self-esteem is heavily invested in their ability to maintain close, harmonious relationships with the people who are important to them. The childbearing period may be one of particular vulnerability because it is a time when women normally expect to feel close to and supported by their romantic partners. A partner's disengagement at this time may be particularly demoralizing. As illustrated in the clinical case, when CBD co-occurs with relationship distress, couples therapy is the treatment of choice. However, couples therapy may be unacceptable to nondepressed partners who have difficulty seeing the relevance of their relationship to their partners' depression (Emanuels-Zuurveen & Emmelkamp, 1996). In these situations, an attachment framework used within the context of individual therapy can help women with CBD to understand how specific relationship difficulties may be driving their depression.

NOTE

1. Although all of the empirical literature to date has examined heterosexual women in co-habiting relationships, most of whom were married to the baby's father, there is no reason to assume that the conceptualization of PPD that I present here would not apply also to women in lesbian relationships and possibly even to single mothers.

REFERENCES

Ainsworth, M., Blehar, M., Waters, E., & Wall, S. (1968). *Patterns of attachment: A psychological study of the strange situation.* Hillsdale, NJ: Erlbaum.

Atkinson, L., Paglia, A., Coolbear, J., Niccols, A., Parker, K. C. H., & Guger, S. (2000). Attachment security: A meta-analysis of maternal mental health correlates. *Clinical Psychology Review, 20,* 1019-1040.

Bagedahl-Strindlund, M., & Ruppert, S. (1998). Parapartum mental illness: A long-term follow-up study. *Psychopathology, 31,* 250-259.

Ballard, C. G., Davis, R., Cullen, P. C., Mohan, R. N., & Dean, C. (1994). Prevalence of postnatal psychiatric morbidity in mothers and fathers. *British Journal of Psychiatry, 164,* 782-788.

Bartholomew, K. (1990). Avoidance of intimacy: An attachment perspective. *Journal of Personal and Social Relationships, 7,* 147-178.

Beck, C. T. (1998). The effects of postpartum depression on child development: A meta-analysis. *Archives of Psychiatric Nursing, 12,* 12-20.

Bowlby, J. (1969). *Attachment and loss Vol. 1: Attachment.* New York: Basic Books.

Bowlby, J. (1973). *Attachment and loss Vol. 2: Separation, anxiety, and anger.* New York: Basic Books.

Bowlby, J. (1980). *Attachment and loss Vol. 3: Loss.* New York: Basic Books.

Burke, K., Burke, J., Regier, D., & Rae, D. (1990). Age of onset of selected mental disorders in five community populations. *Archives of General Psychiatry, 47,* 511-518.

Cooper, P. J., & Murray, L. (1995). Course and recurrence of postnatal depression: Evidence for the specificity of the diagnostic concept. *British Journal of Psychiatry, 166,* 191-195.

Cox, J., Connor, Y., & Kendell, R. (1982). Prospective study of the psychiatric disorders of childbirth. *British Journal of Psychiatry, 140,* 111-117.

Emanuels-Zuurveen, L., & Emmelkamp, P. M. G. (1996). Individual behavioural-cognitive therapy v. marital therapy for depression in maritally distressed couples. *British Journal of Psychiatry, 169,* 181-188.

Gotlib, I. H., Whiffen, V. E., Wallace, P. M., & Mount, J. H. (1991). A prospective investigation of postpartum depression: Factors involved in onset and recovery. *Journal of Abnormal Psychology, 100,* 122-132.

Harris, B., Fung, H., Johns, S., Kologlu, M., Bhatti, R., McGregor, A. M., Richards, C. J., & Hall, R. (1989). Transient post-partum thyroid dysfunction and postnatal depression. *Journal of Affective Disorders, 17,* 243-249.

Hazan, C., & Shaver, P. (1987). Romantic love conceptualized as an attachment process. *Journal of Personality and Social Psychology, 52,* 511-524.

Hunsley, J., Lee, C. M., & Aubry, T. (1999). Who uses psychological services in Canada? *Canadian Psychology, 40,* 232-240.

Jack, D. C. (1991). *Silencing the self: Women and depression.* Cambridge, MA: Harvard University Press.

Johnson, S. M., Makinen, J. A., & Millikin, J. W. (2001). Attachment injuries in couples: A new perspective on impasses in couples therapy. *Journal of Marital and Family Therapy, 27,* 145-155.

Johnson, S. M., & Whiffen, V. E. (1999). Made to measure: Adapting emotionally focused couples therapy to partners' attachment styles. *Clinical Psychology: Science & Practice, 6,* 366-381.

Johnson, S. M., & Whiffen, V. E. (in press). *Attachment: A guide for couple and family interventions.* New York: Guilford.

Marks, M., Wieck, A., Checkley, S., & Kumar, C. (1996). How does marriage protect women with histories of affective disorder from post-partum relapse? *British Journal of Medical Psychology, 69,* 329-342.

Martinez, R., Johnston-Robledo, I., Ulsh, H. M., & Chrisler, J. C. (2000). Singing "the baby blues": A content analysis of popular press articles about postpartum affective disturbances. *Women & Health, 31,* 37-56.

Miller, J. B. (1986). *Toward a new psychology of women.* Boston: Beacon Press.

Neddelbladt, P., Uddenberg, N., & Englesson, I. (1985). Marital disharmony four and a half years postpartum. *Acta Psychiatrica Scandinavica, 71,* 392-401.

Nicolson, P. (1998). *Postnatal depression: Psychology, science and the transition to motherhood.* New York: Routledge.

O'Hara, M. W., Schlechte, J. A., Lewis, D. A., & Varner, M. W. (1991). Controlled prospective study of postpartum mood disorders: Psychological, environmental, and hormonal variables. *Journal of Abnormal Psychology, 100,* 1-11.

O'Hara, M. W., & Swain, A. M. (1996). Rates and risks of postpartum depression: A meta-analysis. *International Review of Psychiatry, 8,* 37-54.

Regier, D., Boyd, J., Burke, J., Rae, D., Myers, J., Kramer, M., Robins, L., George, L., Karno, M., & Locke, B. (1988). One month prevalence of mental disorders in the United States. *Archives of General Psychiatry, 45,* 977-986.

Swendsen, J. D., & Mazure, C. M. (2000). Life stress as a risk factor for postpartum depression: Current research and methodological issues. *Clinical Psychology: Science and Practice, 7,* 17-31.

Teasdale, J. D., Segal, Z. V., Williams, J. M. G., Ridgeway, V. A., Soulsby, J. M., & Lau, M. A. (2000). Prevention of relapse/recurrence in major depression by mindfulness-based cognitive therapy. *Journal of Consulting and Clinical Psychology, 68,* 615-623.

Thompson, J. M., Whiffen, V. E., & Blain, M. D. (1995). Depressive symptoms, sex, and perception of intimate relationships. *Journal of Social and Personal Relationships, 12,* 49-66.

Vandell, D. L., Hyde, J. S., Plant, E. A., & Essex, M. J. (1997). Fathers and "others" as infant-care providers: Predictors of parents' emotional well-being and marital satisfaction. *Merrill-Palmer Quarterly, 43*, 361-385.

Whiffen, V. E. (1992). Is postpartum depression a distinct diagnosis? *Clinical Psychology Review, 12*, 485-508.

Whiffen, V. E., & Gotlib, I. H. (1989a). Stress and coping in maritally distressed and nondistressed couples. *Journal of Social and Personal Relationships, 6*, 327-344.

Whiffen, V., & Gotlib, I. (1989b). Infants of postpartum depressed mothers: Temperament and cognitive status. *Journal of Abnormal Psychology, 98*, 274-279.

Whiffen, V., & Gotlib, I. (1993). Comparison of postpartum and non-postpartum depression: Clinical presentation, psychiatric history, and psycho-social functioning. *Journal of Consulting and Clinical Psychology, 61*, 485-494.

Whiffen, V. E., & Johnson, S. M. (1998). An attachment theory framework for the treatment of childbearing depression. *Clinical Psychology: Science and Practice, 5*, 478-493.

Whiffen, V. E., Kallos-Lilly, A. V., & MacDonald, B. J. (2001). Depression and attachment in couples. *Cognitive Therapy and Research, 25*, 421-434.

Whisman, M. (1999). Marital dissatisfaction and psychiatric disorders: Results from the National Comorbidity Study. *Journal of Abnormal Psychology, 108*, 701-706.

Wisner, K., Perel, J., Peindl, K., Hanusa, B., Findling, R., & Rapport, D. (2001). Prevention of recurrent postpartum depression: A randomized clinical trial. *Journal of Clinical Psychiatry, 62*, 82-86.

Zelkowitz, P., & Milet, T. (1996). Postpartum psychiatric disorders: Their relationship to psychological adjustment and marital satisfaction in the spouses. *Journal of Abnormal Psychology, 105*, 281-285.

Coping with Distress During Perimenopause

Paula S. Derry

SUMMARY. Psychotherapists working with midlife women are likely to encounter perimenopause-related concerns and can play an important role in helping women to cope with distress. In this paper I provide an overview of what perimenopause is, the broad range of concerns that therapists might encounter, and issues related to coping. Perimenopause, the transition leading to and surrounding menopause, has biological and psychosociocultural features. Midlife women may be concerned about physically distressing symptoms, mood changes of uncertain origin, or adult-developmental issues that become entwined with perimenopause. A careful individualized assessment is important, and psychotherapists should address physical experiences along with the psychological interpretations and sociocultural experiences that influence meaning and coping strategies. Responses to uncertainty, negative attitudes toward aging and menopause, and catastrophizing self-statements may be important. *[Article copies available for a fee from The Haworth Document Delivery Service: 1-800-HAWORTH. E-mail address: <docdelivery@haworthpress.com> Website: <http://www.HaworthPress.com> © 2004 by The Haworth Press, Inc. All rights reserved.]*

Paula S. Derry, PhD, is a health psychologist who practices independently in Baltimore, MD. She conducts workshops and provides consultation about menopause and perimenopause for midlife women and health professionals. She has published and presented papers on her theoretical research and analysis of a range of topics that pertain to menopause and perimenopause.

Address correspondence to: Paula S. Derry, PhD, 4811 Crowson Ave., Baltimore, MD 21212 (E-mail: pderry@bcpl.net).

[Haworth co-indexing entry note]: "Coping with Distress During Perimenopause." Derry, Paula S. Co-published simultaneously in *Women & Therapy* (The Haworth Press, Inc.) Vol. 27, No. 3/4, 2004, pp. 165-177; and: *From Menarche to Menopause: The Female Body in Feminist Therapy* (ed: Joan C. Chrisler) The Haworth Press, Inc., 2004, pp. 165-177. Single or multiple copies of this article are available for a fee from The Haworth Document Delivery Service [1-800-HAWORTH, 9:00 a.m. - 5:00 p.m. (EST). E-mail address: docdelivery@haworthpress.com].

http://www.haworthpress.com/store/product.asp?sku=J015
© 2004 by The Haworth Press, Inc. All rights reserved.
10.1300/J015v27n03_12

KEYWORDS. Perimenopause, menopause, coping, midlife

Therapists working with midlife women are likely to encounter perimenopause-related issues. Women may have distressing symptoms or experiences associated with perimenopause or may be uncertain about whether or not their distress is related to this transition. Possible areas of concern span a wide range from uncomfortable physical symptoms to adult-developmental issues. Clients might be anxious because they lack basic information about what is expected/normal during the transition to menopause, because they seek information and find that different sources contradict each other, or because their experience differs from that attributed to perimenopause by their physicians or friends. Symptoms such as hot flashes might be distressing. Clients might wonder whether their moodiness, anxiety, or insomnia is caused by hormonal changes rather than by personal issues and stressors, or they may be certain that this is the case. A wide range of personal issues might become conflated with menopause and aging, as when a woman's response to the end of a relationship or loss of a job is colored by fear that she may never have another chance because she feels old. To develop and maintain a positive self-concept as a midlife woman, a woman might want to sort out what it means to her, if anything, to be perimenopausal, or to separate her own experience from the messages given to her by physicians, advertisements, and friends. A woman to whom menopause is no big deal, or who has a positive experience, might find that her experience is not validated by what she reads or hears others say. Clients might struggle with making decisions about using hormone replacement therapy (HRT) or agreeing to invasive medical procedures such as D & C or hysterectomy.

Psychotherapists who are not physicians can play a role in helping clients to cope with all of these sources of distress. Therapists can provide basic information about the normal course of menopause or direct clients to such information. They can help clients sort their feelings about confusing issues such as decision-making about HRT. They can make suggestions about coping with signs/symptoms. They can be alert to inquiring whether symptoms such as hot flashes might be contributing to moodiness or insomnia, or whether concerns elicited by menopause, such as signs of aging in the body, might have become interwoven with adult-developmental issues such as developing a midlife self-concept. They can assist clients to hear their internal voices as to what their own experience is and to separate that voice from cultural messages.

WHAT IS PERIMENOPAUSE?

All human females naturally stop menstruating during midlife. Menopause is defined retroactively only after a woman has not had a period for 12 months because most women skip periods for amounts of time less than a year before menopause is reached. Perimenopause, the transition that leads to and surrounds menopause, is defined by the World Health Organization (WHO Scientific Group, 1996) as the endocrinological, biological, and clinical features that lead directly to menopause and the first year after periods cease. We now know that perimenopause is important because this (rather than after menopause) is when distressing symptoms are most likely to occur. However, paradoxically, the perimenopause remains ill defined. Professionals disagree about what perimenopause is, when it begins and ends, or exactly what its associated symptoms are. This is because, although we have learned a lot in recent years, much remains unknown about the underlying physiology of the menopause process. In addition, perimenopause is variable: some women don't appear to have any transition between regular periods and menopause, whereas others transition for many years; some women report many symptoms, whereas others are not aware of any; and the meaning of perimenopause varies from catastrophic loss of youth, to a profound inner journey, to wisdom, to nothing at all.

Why women have a menopause is unknown, notwithstanding the strong opinions on the matter held by many professionals. This is not surprising because we also don't know why only women (along with monkeys and apes) menstruate and other mammals do not (Nelson, 1999). As far as we know, humans (and here we differ even from nonhuman primates) are the only mammals that have a complete shutdown of the reproductive system that occurs in midlife, is universal, and is under genetic control (Pavelka & Fedigan, 1991). For reasons we don't know, humans are genetically programmed to have a postreproductive period before old age while they are healthy and, at least among modern hunter/gatherers (e.g., Hawkes, O'Connell, & Burton Jones, 1997; Lee, 1985), important members of their social groups. This might logically imply that menopause is as natural as pregnancy and puberty. Yet the dominant theory of menopause, the biomedical model, presupposes that menopause is abnormal or unhealthy (MacPherson, 1981; Voda, 1992, 1994). Biomedically oriented professionals disagree about wherein lies the unhealthiness. Concepts of what is unhealthy have changed over time; however, the underlying presupposition of unhealthiness does not change (Voda, 1992). Many authors (e.g., Martin, 1992) have pointed out that scientific descriptions of menopause are far from neutral. The ovaries along with other body parts are said to "atrophy," become "senile," and in other ways break down and stop working properly. Some professionals define menopause as a disease of an endocrine organ. Others assert that menopause is "perfectly natural" but nonetheless results in chronic illnesses such as heart, brain, and bone disease because it is a consequence or even an accelerator of aging.

If, in the biomedical viewpoint, menopause is the failure of an aging reproductive system, then perimenopause amounts to the process of breakdown. Perimenopause begins when the reproductive system begins working "improperly," that is, when menstrual periods become irregular or underlying hormonal patterns change from those typical of younger women. Bodily experiences associated with perimenopause such as irregular periods are therefore "symptoms" (p. 7) that require "diagnosis" (p. 6) and possible "treatment" (p. 5) (North American Menopause Society, 2000) rather than, for example, "signs" or "experiences." Compare this to adolescence, where menstrual irregularity is common but not considered a "symptom," or pregnancy, in which "morning sickness" is not a diagnostic sign of illness. Some women do have distressing symptoms during perimenopause. For example, some bleeding changes require medical evaluation, and sometimes hot flashes are severe. However, extreme symptoms are often described to midlife women as though they defined what is common or expected (Voda, 1994).

The perimenopause is often defined as having begun when menstrual periods start to change. However, some women have hot flashes while their periods are still regular; perimenopause is therefore sometimes defined as beginning when symptoms such as hot flashes begin. Because after menopause a hormone called follicle-stimulating hormone (FSH) is present in greater amounts and estrogen levels are lower, it has often been assumed that during the transition to menopause FSH is rising and estrogen is declining. However, although much remains unknown about changes in underlying hormones, the known data do not fit any simple model. FSH can be elevated during one month and not the next; and hot flashes can occur with nonelevated FSH levels, and regular menstrual cycles can be maintained with elevated levels (Prior, 1998). Estrogen levels can be unchanged or elevated rather than low (Prior, 1998). Menstrual periods and hormone levels are often described as being relatively regular until the changes that lead to menopause begin. However, it has also become clear that some changes can be found beginning in a woman's 30s. The quality of periods may change (e.g., how heavy, number of days between periods, number of days of flow), often before periods are frankly irregular or skipped (Mitchell, Woods, & Mariella, 2000). Hormones, such as FSH and estrogen, may also change beginning in the 30s (Prior, 1998). Some clinicians regard these changes as earlier phases of the menopausal transition (e.g., Mitchell, Woods, & Mariella, 2000). Midlife women may be encouraged to look for associated symptoms earlier and earlier (e.g., Goldstein & Ashnet, 1998). However, if changes beginning in the mid-30s count as perimenopause, then the transition to menopause can occur over some 15-20 years, whereas relatively regular menstruation occurs for approximately 20 years, and periods can be relatively irregular up to 8 years after puberty (Treloar, Boynton, Behn, & Brown, 1967). Instead of thinking in terms of an aging reproductive system, therapists could emphasize that there is a life course to menstrual cycles. Which of the changes that occur throughout the life course directly lead to menopause is still unclear.

Menopause is not a purely physiological process. Meaning is attributed to menopause itself and to related symptoms and discomforts. Older stereotypes are that women become mentally unhinged after menopause or lose their femininity, as stated perhaps most infamously by the gynecologist Robert Wilson

(1966) when he wrote that menopausal women "witness the death of their own womanhood" (p. 15) and suffer "the horror of this living decay" (p. 43). As these older stereotypes became discredited they were replaced by newer stereotypes. Menopausal women fear aging and increased vulnerability to chronic disease and hope to be saved by hormone replacement therapy (HRT) (Kaufert, 1994). Although midlife is a sensible time to review ways to minimize one's risk of chronic disease, the importance of menopause and of HRT are far from clear (see Barrett-Connor & Stuenkel, 1999; Grady & Cummings, 2001; Writing Group for the Women's Health Initiative Investigators, 2002; Yaffe, Sawaya, Lieberburg, & Grady, 1998). Research has failed to confirm the existence of a "menopausal syndrome" or a relationship between menopause and serious depression (see below). However, a newer common wisdom now asserts the existence of a "perimenopausal syndrome" that includes "moodiness" and "forgetfulness" (Goldstein & Ashner, 1998).

Dramatic, extreme portrayals of menopause are not limited to the medical community. What menopause means is generally uncertain and contested in American culture. Menopause is often portrayed as a defining event of midlife, the "beginning of the second half of life." Instead of a harbinger of deterioration, it may conversely be described as a renewal or developmental passage (Weed, 1992). Even feminist writings may portray experiences in universalistic terms, such as that all women react strongly to the end of menstrual cycles or their reproductive ability. However, when asked, individual women report that they experience this bodily reorganization, as they do most other experiences, in a variety of ways. Some find the biomedical model to be an accurate portrayal, others experience a profound spiritual or growth journey, and many others find menopause to have no great significance.

DISTRESS DURING PERIMENOPAUSE

Many distressing symptoms and experiences are said to typify the perimenopause, but these become less common as perimenopause ends. Menstrual periods change. Periods with clots, very heavy flow, or very frequent flow tend to be especially worrisome, and unpredictable periods may be annoying or distressing. Vaginal changes ("atrophy") may make intercourse painful. Hot flashes may appear. A hot flash is a sensation of heat, sometimes accompanied by visible reddening or sweating, which has physiological reality (i.e., peripheral body temperature, often measured in the finger, rises). The majority of women rate flashes as creating mild to moderate discomfort and cope well with them, but for some women they are major sources of distress. Flashes become more likely in the years preceeding, and less likely within a few years after, menopause. They vary in frequency, intensity, meaning, and the amount of distress they cause. For some women the flash is purely a feeling of heat; some women report heat with other associated sensations such as a racing heart, nausea, and aura; and for other women cognitions and feelings such as anxiety and catastrophic thoughts accompany the flash.

Perimenopausal women also commonly report other experiences. Many of these changes, such as insomnia, mood changes, memory changes, sexual changes, weight gain, and fatigue, can occur during many different life stages, so it is perhaps not surprising that there is ambiguity and disagreement about when these are related directly to the hormonal changes of perimenopause. Reported mood changes may range from depression and anxiety to irritability. A woman may feel depressed, exhausted/weak, or not able to cope, or she may experience odd memory problems, especially with retrieving words, or sleep problems. Anxiety may be primary, and generalized anxiety may wash over her. Some women wonder whether their productive life is over, and they fear that they may never function well again. Women may or may not feel an inner certainty that these experiences are caused by menopause. Other changes are also reported, such as heart palpitations, headaches, and joint pain; Cobb (1993) included over 100 items in her list of symptoms reported by midlife women.

In formal studies researchers have found that only bleeding changes, hot flashes, and vaginal changes are more common in perimenopausal and/or menopausal, as compared with premenopausal, women (e.g., Holte, 1992; Kaufert, Gilbert, & Tate, 1992). Apart from these changes, symptoms (including affective changes) do not become more common or form a syndrome (i.e., co-occur) as a function of menopause status, although it is possible that future researchers could uncover such evidence or identify subgroups of women for whom such relationships exist. Insomnia becomes more frequent during the 40s and 50s, but appears to be related to many factors, such as depression, anxiety, and hot flashes, with a small possible effect of estrogen levels (Hollander et al., 2001; McKinlay, Brambilla, & Posner, 1992). Premenstrual symptoms may become more common during a woman's 30s or 40s. Well-being is associated with physical symptoms such as hot flashes and psychological variables rather than menopausal status per se. Severe depression is the most researched mood change. As a result, major depressive disorder is no longer attributed to menopause. A series of longitudinal studies (e.g., Kaufert, Gilbert, & Tate, 1992; McKinlay, McKinlay, & Brambilla, 1987) established that clinical levels of depressive symptoms in midlife are more strongly related to history of depression and to life stress (important stressors among midlife women include worry about family members and chronic illnesses such as arthritis) than to menopause status. However, women with a long perimenopause or distressing symptoms such as hot flashes or insomnia are more likely to become depressed (Avis, Brambilla, McKinlay, & Vass, 1994). Some researchers have found greater stress reactivity depending upon menopause status (Saab, Matthews, Stoney, & McDonald, 1989).

A subset of women and their physicians report a direct association between dysphoria and perimenopause. Some women who learn that perimenopause can be associated with a constellation of symptoms such as fatigue, mood changes, problems with memory, and weight gain have an "ah-ha" experience that what they have been feeling has finally been explained in a way that makes sense to them. Some women develop debilitating fatigue or other severe symptoms abruptly during perimenopause. It remains unclear whether these symptoms are primary or secondary to symptoms such as hot flashes and consequent sleep disturbance, or, if directly related to menopause status, what the cause may be. However, for this group, symptoms may remit when they begin HRT. Other women are disappointed when symptoms do not remit with hormone treatment or they develop medication side effects such as depression, headache, or odd bodily sensations.

Women are more likely to feel confused, uncertain, or negative about menopause during the early perimenopause, but, over time, gradually develop a self-image of what it means to be a midife or a menopausal woman and a sense of what the symptoms mean (e.g., Quinn, 1991). The majority of women do not believe that menopause fundamentally changes them, and they greet it with indifference or relief (Avis & McKinlay, 1991). Developmental psychologists (e.g., Notman, 1990) have suggested that women experience an inner reorganization during midife that results in a redefinition of self and other and a greater sense of autonomy and congruence. Menopause may become intertwined with this process of reorganization for some women and symbolize positive or negative aspects of psychological changes. Menopause may also symbolize broader concerns about aging.

COPING WITH DISTRESS DURING PERIMENOPAUSE

Not enough is known about perimenopause to specify definitive approaches to alleviating perimenopausal distress. The discussion below should be read as suggestions about questions to ask, issues to explore, and interventions that might be helpful. The discussion is a mix of research results, professional experience and judgment, and personal insight and speculation.[1]

Coping with perimenopause-related distress begins with a careful, individualized assessment. Changes in periods, hot flashes, vaginal changes, PMS-like symptoms: Which of these is a woman experiencing? Is distress directly due to the physical experience, as when long-term or severe hot flashes are intolerable or result in insomnia, fatigue, or depression? Or might distress be influenced by a woman's interpretation of her bodily experiences, as when she does not attempt to cope with hot flashes that embarrass her at work or indicate to her that she is aging? For ambiguous symptoms such as mood and memory changes, does the woman have, somehow, an inner certainty that these changes are hormonal, "not her," that they have arisen abruptly and for no reason, or some other experience that leads her to believe that these are best understood as being "purely physical"? Have they started at the same time that menstrual flow has changed or hot flashes have arrived or become intolerable? Or might a woman be overestimating the likelihood that her symptoms are due to perimenopause as opposed to life stress or developmental issues, because of cultural stereotypes or personal perceptions? How severe are the symptoms: Do they interfere with daily life and cause intense distress, or are they less intense? Do they cause distress because of fears about what they might mean or assumptions about what they do mean? For example, is a memory problem severe enough to interfere with functioning, a source of embarrassment at work, or of minor practical import but worrisome because it raises the specter of Alzheimer's disease? Distressing symptoms should be situated within the woman's life: the overall picture of her concerns, coping strategies, and the messages she is getting from physicians, advertisements, family, and friends.

Coping with perimenopausal distress, perhaps like any coping, is likely to be facilitated by a positive self-concept and sense of mastery, a positive regard for and comfort with one's body, a positive concept of one's life stage, as well as accurate information about health problems and health-promoting practices. Because many interventions seem to work for some women but not others or for some symptoms but not others, clinical interventions and coping strategies might best be thought of as provisional. A woman should take the stance that she, alone or with a health provider, will try out strategies until she finds those that work for her.

For symptoms that are severe, distressing, or disruptive, a woman may decide to seek a hormone medication. Medication is useful for severe hot flashes, and insomnia may improve. A woman who feels unwell or dysphoric, especially if she also has hot flashes or an inner certainty that hormonal changes are to blame, may seek medication. For perimenopausal women, hormone replacement therapy (HRT), birth control pills, and progesterone have all been prescribed. Alternatively, a woman may seek a complementary practitioner, such as an acupuncturist or a homeopathic physician. Rather than consulting a practitioner, a woman may cope on her own with any of a variety of self-help techniques; for example, for hot flashes, women could dress in layers so that some clothing can be removed when hot, take vitamin E, and use self-monitoring to discover personal triggers. Information about self-help, complementary, and medical options are available in many popular and professional books. For dysphoric symptoms, behavioral interventions such as an exercise program, dietary changes, nurturing oneself, and relaxation might be beneficial. It is important both to validate a woman's experience and to encourage her to reevaluate her experience. For example, a woman may be encouraged to take an active stance to control her negative moods even though she is certain that her dysphoria is caused by hormonal changes. A woman with negative attitudes toward menopause may be asked to list positive aspects of the transition.

Uncertainty and unpredictability are generalized stressors associated with perimenopause. Anxiety might be lower if a woman expects her menstrual cycles to change, has basic guidelines about when these changes might or might not indicate a medical problem, has basic information about what uncomfortable bodily experiences/symptoms might arise during this time, and knows about ways to alleviate distress. Sometimes there is no way of knowing definitely whether distress is due to perimenopause. It may also be useful to explore why uncertainty is uncomfortable. Is this due to a generalized sense that one should be in control of oneself or of one's body, fear that unacceptable experiences will result (as when unpredictable periods or hot flashes create embarrassing situations), or a sense that "menopause shouldn't be happening to me" and that bodily changes are therefore unacceptable? Therapists can recommend that women begin a pleasurable activity such as tennis or yoga in which the body is skilled, or talk with other women about which experiences are common or transient. Anticipating problematic situations may also be useful, as in role-playing responses to anticipated embarrassing situations or always being equipped with tampons and pads. Self-monitoring regimens to track bodily experiences help restore a sense of control and a sense of living in one's body.

We don't know why, but women with negative attitudes toward menopause and aging are more likely to develop hot flashes or depression (e.g., Avis, Crawford, & McKinlay, 1997). Negative expectations about menopause and aging may undercut coping by magnifying distress or discouraging a woman from developing active coping strategies. Psychotherapists can encourage clients to examine negative attitudes, especially those that undercut self-esteem or hope for the future or encourage catastrophic interpretations of bodily experiences. Clinicians can challenge cultural messages that menopause and aging are sad stories about the loss of physical attractiveness, health, cognitive abilities, and social possibilities. Specific exercises, such as describing older women that a client admires or role-playing overcoming a social obstacle to reaching a goal, may be useful. Therapists should encourage clients to seek social support (see Koch and Mansfield, this volume). Cognitive/behavioral factors have been largely unexplored in research, except in small studies of hot flashes and distress. Based on these studies (e.g., Hunter & Liao, 1996; Kittell, Mansfield, & Voda, 1998; Reynolds, 1997) therapists might suggest: relaxation, deep abdominal breathing, role-playing potentially problematic social situations (including stress associated with a social mandate to conceal discomfort), and reframing negative cognitions (especially catastrophic cognitions that hot flashes will be unbearable, last forever, or lead to humiliation).

The psychological meaning of dysphoric experiences needs to be explored carefully, as at any other life stage. Many of the symptoms attributed to perimenopause are also typical of stress. Menopause occurs in a context of personal developmental changes, changes in the family and social situation, and internal reevaluation; life experiences and internal processes combine to produce psychological maturation and personality change (Notman, 1990). Any transition may involve a process of initial confusion or sense of loss, then psychological reevaluation and reorganization, then a final integration. A sense of loss may be one step in a longer process leading to reorganization. Unwillingness to experience the process of transition may be associated with feelings of "being stuck" or dysphoric. It is possible that a subset of perimenopausal women are distressed because they are in a conflict about a developmental transition or because their need to go inward is unacceptable to them for reasons such as fear of aging, distressing memories of one's family of origin, or because they are simply too busy to take the time to explore their internal world.

A KALEIDOSCOPE OF EXPERIENCES

I will close with a portrayal of the variety of experiences possible even for one symptom alone, the hot flash. Esther enjoyed her hot flashes. For the first time in her life, she had times when she wasn't cold in winter. Jane sent her elementary-aged children off to school one warm autumn day without their jackets, only realizing after they left that the day wasn't warm, she had had a hot flash. Marilyn began flashing at age 47. "No big deal. They're kind of interesting." However, when she was still flashing 3 years later, she was at her wits' end. She couldn't take the discomfort, distress, and interrupted sleep for one more day. Theresa found that she would begin flashing in the middle of giving lectures to her college undergraduate class. She turned red, sweaty, dizzy, and anxious, and felt unable to concentrate. "This is completely inappropriate and unacceptable. It has to stop." Carol dreaded her hot flashes. She felt overwhelmed by an intense feeling of heat, like she was trapped inside a burning building, and also nauseous, weak, anxious, and depressed. Hormone medication was a lifesaver. Betty decided to use hormones for her hot flashes. She had a toddler who didn't sleep through the night, she was already waking up during the night, and couldn't afford to lose any more sleep. Marilyn had intense feelings of heat that woke her up at night. Her doctor told her that she was not perimenopausal because her periods were still regular and she was too young. She felt he was not taking her report of her experience seriously. Amber somehow connected the discomfort of hot flashes with other experiences of her body being very sensitive, such as a strong reaction to medications and trouble coming out of anesthesia after dental work. Nancy developed hot flashes after giving birth to her first baby at age 41. She had been having them on and off ever since. Renee began flashing at age 47. "Oh, no. How many years will this go on? Will it get worse and worse? Will I be able to take it?" However, she found that the flashes were annoying but manageable. They lasted for about a year and then stopped. Mary had been waking in the middle of the night, with a shock of anxiety jarring her body. She wondered what threatened her. However, when she focused more closely on her body when this happened, she realized that the shock felt very physical, and right after it she felt warm. She wasn't anxious; she was having a hot flash. Anne found hot flashes extremely uncomfortable. However, when she focused more closely on what she was feeling, she realized that it wasn't the sensation of heat that bothered her. It was that she felt clenched up, the way she did when she was anxious. She found it helpful, when flashing, to remind herself, "This is a hot flash, it will pass soon" while relaxing her body into the flash. Margot felt distressed with every occurrence of a hot flash. However, when she stopped to pay attention to what was going through her mind and body while she flashed, she found herself tensing her body, resisting the flash, and feeling resentful that this was happening to her. "I'm too young for this. This is uncomfortable, and that stinks. It shouldn't be happening to me. I'll probably be flashing for the rest of my life." She coped by stiffening her body and waiting for it to be all over. She decided she did not want to use a hormone medication, and experimented instead with slow, deep, abdominal breathing and self-talk that reassured her that the flash would soon end, that it was okay to flash, and that she could manage it.

CONCLUSION

Psychotherapists should have basic knowledge about the many ways that perimenopause may be related to distress during midlife. Clinicians should be proactive in asking clients whether distress may be menopause-related and prepared to offer clients help in coping. Although it is important for psychotherapists to have specific information about perimenopause and about techniques to manage distressing symptoms, general principles of therapy also remain important. An individual assessment is crucial and symptoms must be understood with reference to personality and personal meaning, situated within the overall life course, and understood with reference to the social context.

NOTE

1. A resource list I have compiled with bibliographies for professionals, readings to recommend to midlife women, suggestions for specific interventions such as self-monitoring instruments, and other materials is available upon request. Make request via e-mail to <pderry@bcpl.net>.

REFERENCES

Avis, N., Brambilla, D., McKinlay, S., & Vass, K. (1994). A longitudinal analysis of the association between menopause and depression. *Annals of Epidemiology, 4,* 214-219.

Avis, N., Crawford, S., & McKinlay, S. (1997). Psychosocial, behavioral, and health factors related to menopause symptomatology. *Women's Health, 3,* 102-120.

Avis, N., & McKinlay, S. (1991). A longitudinal analysis of women's attitudes toward the menopause. *Maturitas, 13,* 65-79.

Barrett-Connor, E., & Stuenkel, C. (1999). Hormones and heart disease in women: Heart and estrogen/progestin replacement study in perspective. *Journal of Clinical Endocrinology and Metabolism, 84,* 1848-1853.

Cobb, J. (1993). *Understanding menopause.* New York: Penguin.

Goldstein, S., & Ashner, L. (1998). *Could it be . . . perimenopause?* New York: Little, Brown.

Grady, D., & Cummings, S. (2001). Postmenopausal hormone therapy for prevention of fractures: How good is the evidence? *Journal of the American Medical Association, 285,* 2909-2910.

Hawkes, K., O'Connell, J., & Burton Jones, N. (1997). Hadza women's time allocation, offspring provisioning, and the evolution of long postmenopausal life spans. *Current Anthropology, 38,* 551-577.

Hollander, L., Freeman, E., Sammel, M., Berlin, J., Grisso, J., & Battistini, M. (2001). Sleep quality, estradiol levels, and behavioral factors in late reproductive women. *Obstetrics & Gynecology, 98,* 391-397.

Holte, A. (1992). Influences of natural menopause on health complaints. *Maturitas, 14,* 127-141.

Hunter, M., & Liao, K. (1996). Evaluation of a four-session cognitive-behavioral intervention for menopausal hot flushes. *British Journal of Health Psychology, 1,* 113-125.

Kaufert, P. (1994). A health and social profile of the menopausal woman. *Experimental Gerontology, 29,* 343-350.

Kaufert, P., Gilbert, P., & Tate, R. (1992). The Manitoba project: A reexamination of the link between menopause and depression. *Maturitas, 14,* 143-155.

Kittell, L., Mansfield, P., & Voda, A. (1998). Keeping up appearances: The basic social process of the menopausal transition. *Qualitative Health Research, 8,* 618-633.

Koch, P. B., & Mansfield, P. K. (2004). Facing the unknown: Social support during the menopausal transition. *Women & Therapy, 27*(3/4), 179-193.

Lee, R. (1985). Work, sexuality, and aging among !Kung women. In J. Brown & V. Kerns (Eds.), *In her prime* (pp. 23-35). South Hadley, MA: Bergin and Garvey.

MacPherson, K. (1981). Menopause as disease: The social construction of a metaphor. *Advances in Nursing Science, 3,* 95-113.

Martin, E. (1992). *The woman in the body.* Boston: Beacon Press.

McKinlay, J., McKinlay, S., & Brambilla, D. (1987). The relative contributions of endocrine changes and social circumstances to depression in middle-aged women. *Journal of Health and Social Behavior, 28,* 345-356.

McKinlay, S., Brambilla, D., & Posner, J. (1992). The normal menopause transition. *Maturitas, 14,* 103-115.

Mitchell, E., Woods, N., & Mariella, A. (2000). Three stages of the menopausal transition from the Seattle Midlife Women's Health Study: Toward a more precise definition. *Menopause, 7,* 334-349.

Nelson, R. (1999). *An introduction to behavioral endocrinology.* Sunderland, MA: Sinauer.

North American Menopause Society. (2000). Clinical challenges of perimenopause: Consensus opinion of The North American Menopause Society. *Menopause, 7,* 5-13.

Notman, M. (1990). Menopause and adult development. *Annals of the New York Academy of Sciences, 592,* 149-155.

Pavelka, M., & Fedigan, L. (1991). Menopause: A comparative life history perspective. *Yearbook of Physical Anthropology, 34,* 13-38.

Prior, J. (1998). Perimenopause: The complex endocrinology of the menopausal transition. *Endocrine Reviews, 19,* 397-428.

Quinn, A. (1991). A theoretical model of the perimenopausal process. *Journal of Nurse-Midwifery, 36,* 25-29.

Reynolds, F. (1997). Psychological responses to menopausal hot flushes: Implications of a qualitative study for counselling interventions. *Counselling Psychology Quarterly, 10,* 309-321.

Saab, P., Matthews, K., Stoney, C., & McDonald, R. (1989). Premenopausal and postmenopausal women differ in their cardiovascular and neuroendocrine responses to behavioral stressors. *Psychophysiology, 26,* 270-280.

Treloar, A., Boynton, R., Behn, B., & Brown, B. (1967). Variation of the human menstrual cycle through reproductive life. *International Journal of Fertility, 12,* 77-126.

Voda, A. (1992). Menopause: A normal view. *Clinical Obstetrics and Gynecology, 35,* 923-933.

Voda, A. (1994). Risks and benefits associated with hormonal and surgical therapies for healthy midlife women. *Western Journal of Nursing Research, 16,* 507-523.

Weed, S. (1992). *Menopausal years: The wise woman way.* Woodstock, NY: Ash Tree.

WHO Scientific Group. (1996). *Research on the menopause in the 1990s.* A report of the WHO Scientific Group. Geneva, Switzerland: World Health Organization.

Wilson, R. (1966). *Feminine forever.* New York: Evans.

Writing Group for the Women's Health Initiative Investigators. (2002). Risks and benefits of estrogen plus progestin in healthy postmenopausal women. *Journal of the American Medical Association, 288,* 321-333.

Yaffe, K., Sawaya, G., Lieberburg, I., & Grady, D. (1998). Estrogen therapy in postmenopausal women: Effects on cognitive function and dementia. *Journal of the American Medical Association, 279,* 688-695.

Facing the Unknown:
Social Support
During the Menopausal Transition

Patricia Barthalow Koch
Phyllis Kernoff Mansfield

SUMMARY. Many midlife women are uncertain about the indicators of menopause and how to negotiate the menopausal transition. They need accurate information regarding perimenopause and menopause. They need to learn to cope with their changing bodies, appearance, and sexuality, as well as issues related to aging in a youth-oriented society. To do this, they need to learn how to access and mobilize the informational, emotional, and instrumental support that they need from their existing social networks. They may also have to develop new social networks, as well as develop effective strategies for interacting with supportive professional helpers. In this article, we review the literature on the role of social support in women's health and emphasize the key concerns of women during their menopausal transition. Specific recommendations

Patricia Barthalow Koch is Associate Professor of Biobehavioral Health and Women's Studies at The Pennsylvania State University and Assistant Director of the Tremin Trust Research Program on Women's Health. Phyllis Kernoff Mansfield is Professor of Women's Studies and Health Education at The Pennsylvania State University and Director of the Tremin Trust.

Address correspondence to: Patricia Barthalow Koch, E-304 Henderson Building, The Pennsylvania State University, University Park, PA 16802 (E-mail: p3k@psu.edu).

The authors acknowledge the assistance of Molly Carey and Robert Moody.

[Haworth co-indexing entry note]: "Facing the Unknown: Social Support During the Menopausal Transition." Koch, Patricia Barthalow, and Phyllis Kernoff Mansfield. Co-published simultaneously in *Women & Therapy* (The Haworth Press, Inc.) Vol. 27, No. 3/4, 2004, pp. 179-194; and: *From Menarche to Menopause: The Female Body in Feminist Therapy* (ed: Joan C. Chrisler) The Haworth Press, Inc., 2004, pp. 179-194. Single or multiple copies of this article are available for a fee from The Haworth Document Delivery Service [1-800-HAWORTH, 9:00 a.m. - 5:00 p.m. (EST). E-mail address: docdelivery@haworthpress.com].

10.1300/J015v27n03_13

are made regarding helpful social support strategies and resources for women facing menopause. *[Article copies available for a fee from The Haworth Document Delivery Service: 1-800-HAWORTH. E-mail address: <docdelivery@haworthpress.com> Website: <http://www.HaworthPress.com> © 2004 by The Haworth Press, Inc. All rights reserved.]*

KEYWORDS. Social support, menopause, perimenopause, midlife

By 2020, there will be as many women facing menopause in the United States as there will be women in their childbearing years (United States Department of Commerce, 1998). Menopause has been described as a potential time for both crisis and opportunity (McQuaide, 1996). The physical, emotional, menstrual, and sexual changes that may take place during the years prior to menopause, known as perimenopause, create dual challenges (Kittell, Mansfield, & Voda, 1998). First, women face the unpredictability of menopause-related changes. Second, they have to learn ways to cope with these changes.

Researchers have begun to document the perimenopausal changes that women experience. For example, in the Tremin Trust Research Program on Women's Health, a longitudinal study of the menopausal transition, the majority of women reported physical changes, including weight gain, fatigue, joint pain, and food cravings (Mansfield & Voda, 1997). The bleeding pattern often became shorter, then longer and more variable; bleeding became heavier with gushing and clots (Treloar, 1981; Voda & Mansfield, 1991). In addition, nearly 40% of the women reported sexual changes, including decreasing sexual desire and arousal, engaging in sexual activity less often, and desiring more nongenital touching (Mansfield, Koch, & Voda, 1998). This perimenopausal transition may last up to 11 years, until women reach menopause (the cessation of menses for 12 months) at the average age of 51 (Treloar, 1981).

In order to negotiate this transition, women need support in its many forms: informational, emotional, and instrumental. Although there is a dearth of research on the relationships among various aspects of social support and the menopausal experience, there is research that provides insight into the impact of social support on women's health and well-being.

In this review, we examine the impact of social support on women's health and emphasize the key concerns of women during their menopausal transition. The social support needs of midlife women are described based on research on the menopausal transition. Specific recommendations are made regarding helpful social support strategies and resources for women facing menopause.

SOCIAL SUPPORT

Social support is defined as aid from significant others that is intended to meet the emotional, informational, or instrumental needs of an individual

(Heaney & Israel, 1998). The provision of social support is an important function of social networks, the person-centered webs of social relationships. Social support operates in complex ways and is not fully understood. The buffer theory suggests that social support impacts health by reducing the harmful effects of stress (Schwarzer & Leppin, 1991). On the other hand, social support may directly affect health, independent of stress levels, by bolstering more positive affective states or providing needed information or resources that facilitate positive health practices. Difficulties in studying social support lie in the inconsistencies in conceptualization, which have led to measurement variations.

Social support is identified as being consciously provided by the sender in order to be helpful. Different types of support may be provided by various network members in differing situations (Heaney & Israel, 1998). Informational support is the provision of advice, suggestions, and information that a person can use in addressing problems. To be supportive, information should be provided in an interpersonal context of caring, trust, and respect for each person's right to self-determination. Emotional support is the provision of empathy, love, trust, and caring. Instrumental support is the provision of tangible aid and services that directly assist a person in need.

Women and Social Support

In comparison to men's social networks, women's networks are more variable and serve more functions (Shumaker & Hill, 1991). Throughout the life span, women tend to have more intensive networks than men do. Women cast a wider net of concern, are more responsive to the life events of others, and get involved in more supportive activities. Thus, women are highly likely to be both support providers and support recipients in all forms of help-giving. Their large social networks provide opportunities for support, but can also lead to more demands and depletion of resources (Schwarzer & Leppin, 1991; Shumaker & Hill, 1991). This can result in what has been referred to as the "cost of caring" or "contagion of stress" (Solomon & Rothblum, 1986). In other words, networks can create and exacerbate, as well as relieve, women's stress. A balanced or reciprocal provider-and-recipient relationship has been shown to have a great influence on social support satisfaction for women (Shumaker & Hill, 1991). Therefore, women must learn to be protective of themselves by not overextending their personal resources. In addition, they need to know how to access and mobilize the support that they need.

Social Support and Health

Despite diverse research methodologies, a large body of research has documented a robust relationship between social support, across a variety of support providers, and various physical and mental health outcomes (Primomo,

Yates, & Woods, 1990; Uchino, Cacioppo, & Kiecolt-Glaser, 1996). Lower levels of social support are associated with higher incidences of mortality and morbidity for a wide range of mental and physical diseases. A low level of social support is associated with psychological distress, psychosomatic complaints, and physiological indices of stress (Solomon & Rothblum, 1986). Thus, insufficient social support is a risk factor for poor health. On the other hand, higher levels of social support are associated with improved coping with medical problems, use of preventive health practices, and prevention of stress-induced illnesses (Hurdle, 2001). Having a confiding intimate relationship with another person appears to reduce psychological and somatic distress throughout life, including midlife (Brown, Andrews, Harris, Adler, & Bridge, 1986; Cooke, 1985).

Family, friends, and other members of the social network often play a significant role in how an individual adapts to a chronic illness, such as breast disease, diabetes, or cancer (Primomo, Yates, & Woods, 1990). Greater levels of emotional support from family members to someone who is chronically ill are related to enhanced well-being, less anxiety and depression, better social adjustment, and higher levels of physical functioning. Higher levels of instrumental support are associated with higher self-esteem, better mood, and improved physical recovery. In a study of cancer patients, Dunkel-Schetter (1984) found that emotional and instrumental support provided by family, friends, or health-care personnel were equally helpful. However, informational support was considered more helpful when it came from a health-care provider than from family or friends.

Correlations have also been found between social support and women's reproductive health. For example, perceived prenatal social support has emerged as a predictor of infant birth weight (Da Costa, 2000). Specifically, women who reported less satisfaction with their social support in the second trimester of pregnancy gave birth to infants of lower birth weight. In another study, women who experienced dysmenorrhea had less adequate social support than women who did not report painful menstruation (Whittle, Slade, & Ronalds, 1987). In regard to menopause, women who lack social support are more likely to seek medical care for menopausal complaints than those who have a social support network, including a satisfying relationship with a sexual partner (Montero, Ruiz, & Hernandez, 1993).

WOMEN'S NEEDS
DURING THE MENOPAUSAL TRANSITION

Women's greatest concern about menopause is uncertainty about the indicators of menopause, including what experiences to anticipate, and whether the emotional, menstrual, and other changes they are experiencing are typical of the menopausal transition (Cobb, 1998; Jones, 1994; Lemaire & Lenz,

1995; Mansfield, Theisen, & Boyer, 1992; Walter, 2000). In fact, ignorance of the typical changes that occur during the menopausal transition has been described by women as the worst aspect of their menopausal experience (Mansfield & Jorgensen, 1992).

For many women, menopause is still shrouded in secrecy because there continues to be a reluctance to discuss openly feelings and anxieties beyond superficial menstrual cycle changes and the use of hormone replacement therapy (Walter, 2000). In our society, menopause tends to be framed in a negative, medicalized perspective as a "deficiency disease" (Jones, 1994). This makes it difficult for women to view menopause from a more natural and comprehensive perspective and to explore the psychosocial meanings menopause has for them. Confusing these issues even further is the plethora of conflicting information provided by the media and health-care system.

Lack of Information

Most women lack accurate knowledge about menopause and have difficulty separating myth from fact (Hamburger & Anderson, 1990). Such ignorance needs to be ameliorated because perimenopausal women who are fully informed about and prepared for menopause are more likely than less informed women to approach the transition with less fear and a greater sense of control (Hunter, 1996).

Nevertheless, few women have received detailed information through their schooling regarding menopause (Jones, 1994). Studies indicate that most women have never engaged in informative discussions with their mothers or other older female relatives concerning what to expect, although they wish they had had such discussions (Mansfield & Voda, 1993; Walter, 2000). Most mothers either did not want to discuss menopause or were unavailable when daughters needed their support.

Instead many women turn to their friends or the media to gain information. In one study of perimenopausal women, over one-half (53.7%) had their last conversation about menopause with friends, although many of these conversations made light of menopausal symptoms (Mansfield & Voda, 1993). In another study, over one-third (35%) of midlife women said that they had no one to talk to about menopause (Mansfield, Theisen, & Boyer, 1992). This figure was highest (60%) among those most likely to be going through perimenopause, 46-50-year-old women.

The most common reason why perimenopausal women in the Tremin Women's Health Program visited physicians was to discuss their menstrual cycle changes (Mansfield, Koch, & Voda, 1991). Women also reported visiting physicians to discuss their emotional changes, hot flashes, sexuality, and other body changes. This resulted in over one-third (37%) of these women being placed on hormone replacement therapy (HRT) for their menstrual cycle changes and over three-quarters (78%) given HRT for hot flashes. Although women often rely on physicians for information concerning other aspects of their health, midlife women have reported that they received insufficient or biased information from their physicians regarding menopause (Mansfield & Voda, 1993; Quinio, 1999; Walter, 2000). This has resulted in physicians being identified as the least supportive source of menopausal information for many midlife women, as described below:

> Most MDs "push" hormone treatment and are not willing to listen to my concerns. I feel that they are being swayed by drug companies . . . I feel I get only half the information, half the treatment, and half the follow-up available.

> I asked my doctor if I was experiencing menopause. He said, "Don't concern yourself about that. Women in this state don't have menopause until they are in their 50s." I did not use his services anymore. (Mansfield, Theisen, & Boyer, 1992, pp. 77-78)

In addition, Wilt and Kirk (1995) found that even psychotherapists are hesitant to discuss menopausal issues with their menopausal patients.

Aging and Appearance

As women progress through the menopausal transition, they need to deal with many other midlife issues related, or in addition, to menopause. One of the most difficult is how to accept one's aging in a culture that values youth, particularly in women (Jones, 1994). Women's aging in our culture is fraught with both ageism and sexism (Abu-Laban, 1981; Shaw, 1994). In our youth-oriented culture, growing older may signify a loss of value for a woman that can negatively affect her overall self-esteem (Chrisler & Ghiz, 1993; Pearlman, 1993).

Along with the stigma attached to aging, midlife women must deal with the nearly impossible cultural standards of female attractiveness. Thurau (1996) found that one in five (21%) midlife women could not identify anything attractive about their bodies. Only 16% described themselves as currently being more attractive than they were 10 years ago, whereas 33% felt equally attractive to their more youthful selves. Fully half of the women reported that they were currently less attractive than they had been 10 years earlier. Women worried about appearing old and "drying up." Some of the women's body image concerns are expressed in the following quotes:

> Getting matronly looking, gaining weight, looking thick and losing sexual appeal.

> Fifty is too young to be "old." I fear beginning to look like my mother with a very large stomach! (Mansfield & Voda, 1993, p. 97)

Sexual Changes

Several studies have shown that midlife women report many sexual changes as they experience the menopausal transition (Avis, Stellato, Crawford, Johannes, & Longcope, 2000; Dennerstein, Dudley, & Burger, 2001; Johnson, 1998). In one study, some midlife women reported enjoying sex more (8.7%), easier arousal (8.7%), desiring sex more (7.0%), easier orgasm (6.7%), and engaging in sex more often (4.7%) (Mansfield, Koch, & Voda, 1998). These women attributed their improved sexuality most often to changes in life circumstances (e.g., new partner, more freedom with children leaving home), improved emotional well-being, more positive feelings toward their partner, and improved appearance (Mansfield, Koch, & Voda, 2000).

However, two to three times more women reported declines in their sexual responding, including: desiring sex less (23.1%), engaging in sex less often (20.7%), desiring more nongenital touching (19.7%), more difficult arousal (19.1%), enjoying sex less (15.4%), more difficult orgasm (14.0%), and more pain (10.0%) (Mansfield, Koch, & Voda, 2000). Women were much more likely to attribute declining sexual response to physical changes of menopause than to other factors. Although significant relationships were found between having vaginal dryness and decreased sexual desire and enjoyment, no significant relationships between menopausal status and decreased sexual desire, enjoyment, or more difficulty with orgasm were found (Mansfield, Voda, & Koch, 1995). Other researchers who studied general populations of aging women have found similar results (Avis, Stellato, Crawford, Johannes, & Longcope, 2000; Hawton, Gaith, & Day, 1994).

Rather than menopausal status, context seems to be the critical component of women's sexual expression. For example, most of the Tremin participants described some aspect of intimacy, such as love, closeness, sharing, companionship, affection, and caring, as being the most important aspect of their sexual experience (Koch & Mansfield, 2001/2002). Qualities exhibited by their sexual partners, who most often were the women's husbands, have been found to impact the women's sexual responding significantly (Mansfield, Koch, & Voda, 1998). Specifically, the more love, affection, passion, assertiveness, interest, and equality expressed by the sexual partners, the higher the levels of the women's sexual desire, arousal, frequency, and enjoyment. As one woman described:

> My partner is very accepting about how I feel and what I like and what I don't like even though it changes often. I also appreciate that he doesn't expect me to have an orgasm every time we make love. (Koch & Mansfield, 2001/2002, p. 6)

SOCIAL SUPPORT STRATEGIES

In this section, we are going to make suggestions that can be used by psychotherapists, health-care practitioners, or others to help women develop the social support they need during their menopausal transition. Because midlife is a time of transition in so many ways, women need to learn how to create new meanings for their own lives. Jones (1994) suggested that women learn to embody their lives, i.e., that they become more attuned to their bodies. To do this, women need to know that considerable variation exists in the way women experience menopause, what it means for them, how it affects their bodies and lives, and how they respond to it. They should be encouraged to monitor the changes they are experiencing so that they can discover their own patterns (Cobb, 1998).

With increased informational, emotional, and instrumental support, midlife women will be able to develop a new sense of wisdom, power, vigor, resilience, and a stronger sense of self (Jones, 1994). Women must first become more aware of the importance of social support during this time in their lives. They should assess the support they are currently receiving in order to know how to mobilize the support that they need and find new avenues of support when necessary.

Three basic strategies for improving social support include: enhancing existing social linkages, developing new social networks when needed, and using professional helpers who work with clients to meet their needs (Heaney & Israel, 1998). Women will be best served when there is a strong network of both informal and formal helpers so that each type of helper brings her or his unique skills and strengths to the support process (Heaney & Israel, 1998; Kalbfleisch & Bonnell, 1996).

Enhancing Existing Social Networks

Women report turning to their friends most often for support concerning menopause. Thus, they can be encouraged to share accurate information and delve into all of the issues that surround menopause and aging in discussions with their friends. Guidelines for developing a menopause discussion group are provided by the North American Menopause Society (NAMS), the leading nonprofit organization devoted to promoting women's health during midlife and beyond through an understanding of menopause (Boggs & Rosenthal, 2000). Granville (1990) provided another outline for facilitating a menopause support group. A support group may be organized informally among groups of friends or may become more formal and reach out to women throughout the community. Groups can be started by feminist therapists or peer-run by women themselves.

A list of ongoing menopause discussion groups in the United States and Canada is provided on the NAMS Web site (www.menopause.org). Up-to-date information to be shared through these discussions can be found at this Web site also. NAMS has prepared *The Menopause Guidebook* (2001) that presents menopause basics, including perimenopausal changes, post-menopausal health issues, and menopausal treatment options. A brief list of other helpful written materials is provided at the end of this article.

Although most married women report turning to their husbands as a primary source of support in dealing with many health issues, husbands tend to be less able to offer support when it comes to menopause. In a study of the husbands of participants in the Midlife Women's Health Survey, nearly two-thirds (63.5%) of the men reported that they tried to provide emotional or instrumental support to their wives regarding menopause (Mansfield, Koch, & Gierach, 2003). Yet their support efforts were hampered due to a lack of understanding about menopause and the stresses that they were facing in their own lives, including work, finances, and health problems. For example, over one-fourth (27.6%) of the men said that they knew nothing or nearly nothing about menopause. Furthermore, one-fourth (24.2%) of the husbands believed that their wives' menopausal transition had had an adverse effect on them.

> The primary effect of my wife's transition on me is confusion and trepidation. I do not know what tendencies are just my wife's nature versus the effect of menopause. (Mansfield, Koch, & Gierach, 2003)

These findings underscore the importance of providing better education about menstruation and menopause to both women and men throughout their lives. In addition, more educational and support services need to be offered to midlife men to better prepare them to deal with the transitions that both they and their wives will be going through. Men could be involved with special sessions of menopause discussion and support groups, and menopause workshops could even be offered to couples.

Developing New Social Networks

It has been argued that social support is more effective when it comes from those who are socially similar in values and characteristics and who are facing or have faced similar stressors somewhat successfully (Thoits, 1986). Thus, midlife women may need to broaden their existing social networks to include more individuals who meet these criteria, namely women who are dealing, or have already dealt, with midlife/menopausal issues in helpful, positive, and enhancing ways.

In today's society, the Internet offers instant access to networks that can provide information, emotional, and sometimes even instrumental support. In addition to the NAMS Web site previously discussed, a few other excellent Web sites are briefly described.

A Friend Indeed is a printed and online (www.afriendindeed.ca) newsletter that provides information and support to women in menopause and midlife. It is a respected, woman-centered source of understandable and reliable information about the menopausal transition, independent of any vested interests. While providing up-to-date information on menopausal issues, *A Friend Indeed* also offers two important services. The first service is a set of guidelines for evaluating media reports about menopausal research. The second is a roadmap of "Menopause on the Web: Venturing into Cyberspace," which offers pointers for evaluating online health information.

Menopause Online (www.menopause-online.com) also provides up-to-date, easy to use information to smooth the menopausal transition. In addition, it offers the opportunity to communicate with other women about menopausal issues, including physical, emotional, and sexual changes, treatment options, and alternative therapies. Women can communicate with others through topic-specific bulletin boards or via a live chat room.

The *Power Surge* Web site (www.power-surge.com) describes itself as a powerfully effective support group for women. It strives to create a warm and caring community for women during their menopausal transition. It does this through many means, including weekly "chat" sessions with medical professionals, a message board with a transcript library, and 24-hour online support. Visitors may also engage in interactive conferences with guest experts on different menopausal issues.

Engaging Professional Helpers

Midlife women whose support needs are not being met through other means may engage professional helpers to access the information, counseling, or treatment options that they believe they need. However, women are often dissatisfied with the information and care that their physicians provide regarding menopausal transition (Mansfield & Voda, 1993; Walter, 2000).

Responses from the Midlife Women's Health Survey show that nearly one-half (48%) of the participants who had visited a physician with a menopause-related concern noted that the physician did not provide enough information about menopause, hormone replacement therapy, or alternatives to hormones (Quinio, 1999). In fact, some women believed that they found better information on their own than their practitioner provided to them. Other criticisms included the physician treating menopause as an illness, not spending enough time with the woman during the office visits, not encouraging the woman to make her own decisions, not showing respect or support for the woman, and "pushing hormones." The women themselves were most likely to initiate discussions with their physicians regarding their menstrual cycle and other body changes, hot flashes, incontinence, vaginal dryness, and sexuality issues. On the other hand, physicians were most likely to initiate discussions about cardiovascular disease, osteoporosis, and hormone replacement therapy. The following quote encapsulates midlife women's frustrations:

> Most health-care practitioners know little to nothing about menopause or the five or so years that precede it. Furthermore, they only seem interested in hearing about things/symptoms for which they can prescribe hormones or a hysterectomy. I like my usual health-care practitioner (a woman certified physician assistant). But she's not interested in talking about alternative ways of dealing with menopause other than to "treat" it as an illness. (Quinio, 1999, p. 43)

Traits that the midlife women noted as most helpful about their practitioners included spending time, listening, providing full current information, being supportive and respectful, and allowing the woman make her own decisions (Kittell & Mansfield, 2000; Quinio, 1999) as described below:

> My physician's most helpful trait is his willingness to discuss options, answer any and all questions and give reasons for his opinions. I am satisfied and comfortable with the information I received regarding menopause because he tailored in to MY situation. He took into account my medical history, the medical history of my family, and explained his conclusions in terms of what he recommended for me, yet acknowledged that the decision was mine to make. (Quinio, 1999, p. 38)

It may be a challenge to find a physician who is supportive of exploring all of the options for dealing with menopausal issues. NAMS provides a list on their Web site of recommended menopause health professionals located in the United States and Canada. The Agency for Healthcare Research and Quality provides excellent self-help guidelines for choosing a physician on their Web site (www.ahcpr.gov/consumer/qntascii/qntdr.htm).

A blueprint for offering education and social-psychological support through a menopause clinic is provided by Hamburger and Anderson (1990). They recommend that such a clinic facilitate discussions among groups of four to six women with individual counseling offered to each person. The women should be encouraged to share their experiences and concerns within the permissive and sympathetic atmosphere created in the group. Each woman should also be encouraged to keep a diary of her perimenopausal experiences. A "hot flash line" should be made available for additional staff support. This blueprint can serve as a starting point for establishing a menopause clinic in a local hospital or health center.

There is much psychotherapists can do to help ease the menopausal transition for their midlife clients. Even if perimenopausal symptoms or concerns about menopause are not presenting problems, the therapist may want to assess the client's menopausal status. Issues concerning the client's changing body, appearance, and sexuality could be explored. The therapist could determine the client's need for informational, emotional, or instrumental support in coping with the menopausal transition and suggest strategies for mobilizing that support. The therapist could also provide access to the written and Internet resources noted in this article.

CONCLUSION

To conclude, midlife women are most concerned with the uncertainty of the indicators of menopause and knowing how to negotiate the unknown menopausal experience. They often lack the informational, emotional, and instrumental support that they need. Although little research has been done specifically on the relationships among social support and physical and emotional health during menopausal transition, a large body of research has documented a robust relationship between social support and various physical and mental health outcomes.

Midlife women need accurate information regarding perimenopausal transition and menopause. They also need to learn to cope with their changing appearance and sexuality, as well as issues related to aging in a youth-oriented society (Mansfield & Koch, 1997). To do this, they need to learn how to access and mobilize the informational, emotional, and instrumental support that they need from their existing social networks. They may also have to develop new social networks, as well as implement strategies for interacting with supportive professional helpers.

RECOMMENDED RESOURCES

Written Material

The Boston Women's Health Book Collective. (1998). *Our bodies, ourselves for the new century.* New York: Simon & Schuster.
The Boston Women's Health Book Collective. (1994). *The new ourselves getting older.* New York: Simon & Schuster.
The National Women's Health Network. Pamphlets on menopause issues (e.g., *Menopause, Alternative Therapies, Making Choices About Hormones*). Write to: 514 Tenth Street, Suite 400, Washington, DC 20004 (nominal fee).
Voda, A. (1997). *Menopause, me and you.* Binghamton, NY: Harrington Park Press.

Web Sites

A Friend Indeed (www.afriendindeed.ca); also provides a printed newsletter.
Menopause Online (www.menopause-online.com)
North American Menopause Society (www.menopause.org)
Power Surge (www.power-surge.com)
The Agency for Healthcare Research and Quality (www.ahcpr.gov)

REFERENCES

Abu-Laban, S. M. (1981). Women and aging: A futurist perspective. *Psychology of Women Quarterly, 6*, 85-99.

Avis, N. E., Stellato, M. A., Crawford, S., Johannes, C., & Longcope, C. (2000). Is there an association between menopause status and sexual functioning? *Menopause, 7*, 297-309.

Boggs, P. P., & Rosenthal, M. B. (2000). Helping women help themselves: Developing a menopause discussion group. *Clinical Obstetrics and Gynecology, 43*, 207-212.

Brown, G., Andrews, B., Harris, T., Adler, Z., & Bridge, L. (1986). Social support, self-esteem, and depression. *Psychological Medicine, 16*, 813-831.

Chrisler, J. C., & Ghiz, L. (1993). Body image issues of older women. *Women & Therapy, 14*(1/2), 67-75.

Cobb, J. O. (1998). Reassuring the woman facing menopause: Strategies and resources. *Patient Education and Counseling, 33*, 281-288.

Cooke, D. J. (1985). Social support and stressful life events during mid-life. *Maturitas, 7*, 303-313.

Da Costa, D. M. (2000). A prospective study on the influence of stress, social support, and coping on birth outcomes and depressive symptomology during pregnancy and the postpartum. *Dissertation Abstracts International, 60*(8-B), 4213.

Dennerstein, L., Dudley, E., & Burger, H. (2001). Are changes in sexual functioning during midlife due to aging or menopause? *Fertility and Sterility, 76*, 456-460.

Dunkel-Schetter, C. (1984). Social support in cancer: Findings based on patient interviews and their implications. *Journal of Social Issues, 40*, 77-98.

Granville, G. (1990). Facilitating a menopause support group. *Health Visitor, 63*(3), 82-83.

Hamburger, S., & Anderson, E. R. (1990). The value of education and social-psychological support in a menopause clinic. *Annals of New York Academy of Sciences, 592*, 242-249.

Hawton, K., Gaith, D., & Day, A. (1994). Sexual function in a community sample of middle-aged women with partners: Effects of age, marital, socioeconomic, psychiatric, gynecological, and menopausal factors. *Archives of Sexual Behavior, 23*, 375-395.

Heaney, C. A., & Israel, B. A. (1998). Social networks and social support. In K. Glanz, F. M. Lewis, & B. K. Rimer (Eds.), *Health behavior and health education: Theory, research, and practice* (pp. 179-205). San Francisco: Jossey-Bass.

Hunter, M. (1996). Menopause. In C. Niven & A. Walker (Eds.), *Reproductive potential and fertility control* (pp. 59-76). Oxford: Butterworth-Heinemann.

Hurdle, D. E. (2001). Social support: A critical factor in women's health and health promotion. *Health & Social Work, 26*(2), 72-79.

Johnson, B. K. (1998). A correlational framework for understanding sexuality in women age 50 and older. *Health Care for Women International, 19*, 533-564.

Jones, J. (1994). Embodied meaning: Menopause and the change of life. *Social Work in Health Care, 19*, 44-65.

Kalbfleisch, P. J., & Bonnell, K. H. (1996). Menarche, menstruation, and menopause: The communication of information and social support. In R. L. Parrott & C. M. Condit (Eds.), *Evaluating women's health messages: A resource book* (pp. 265-278). Thousand Oaks, CA: Sage.

Kittell, L. A., & Mansfield, P. K. (2000). What perimenopausal women think about using hormones during menopause. *Women & Health, 30*(4), 77-91.

Kittell, L. A., Mansfield, P. K., & Voda, A. M. (1998). Keeping up appearances: The basic social process of the menopausal transition. *Qualitative Health Research, 8*, 618-633.

Koch, P. B., & Mansfield, P. K. (2001/2002). Women's sexuality as they age: The more things change, the more they stay the same. *SIECUS Report, 30*(2), 5-9.

Lemaire, G. S., & Lenz, E. R. (1995). Perceived uncertainty about menopause in women attending an educational program. *International Journal of Nursing Studies, 32*(1), 39-48.

Mansfield, P. K., & Jorgensen, C. M. (1992). Menstrual pattern changes in middle-aged women. In A. J. Dan & L. L. Lewis (Eds.), *Menstrual health in women's lives* (pp. 213-225). Chicago: University of Illinois Press.

Mansfield, P. K., & Koch, P. B. (1997). Enhancing your sexual response. *Menopause Management, 6*(2), 18C.

Mansfield, P. K., Koch, P. K., & Gierach, G. (2003). Husbands' support of their perimenopausal wives. *Women & Health, 38*, 99-114.

Mansfield, P. K., Koch, P. B., & Voda, A. M. (1991). [Midlife women's interaction with physicians regarding menopause]. Unpublished raw data.

Mansfield, P. K., Koch, P. B., & Voda, A. M. (1998). Qualities midlife women desire in their sexual relationships and their changing sexual response. *Psychology of Women Quarterly, 22*, 285-303.

Mansfield, P. K., Koch, P. B., & Voda, A. M. (2000). Midlife women's attributions for their sexual response changes. *Health Care for Women International, 21*, 543-559.

Mansfield, P. K., Thiesen, S. C., & Boyer, B. (1992). Midlife women and menopause: A challenge for the mental health counselor. *Journal of Mental Health Counseling, 14*(1), 73-83.

Mansfield, P. K., & Voda, A. (1993). From Edith Bunker to the 6:00 news: How and what midlife women learn about menopause. *Women & Therapy, 14*(1/2), 89-104.

Mansfield, P. K., & Voda, A. (1997). Woman-centered information on menopause for health care providers: Findings from the Midlife Women's Health Survey. *Health Care for Women International, 18*, 55-72.

Mansfield, P. K., Voda, A., & Koch, P. K. (1995). Predictors of sexual response changes in heterosexual midlife women. *Health Values, 19*(1), 10-20.

McQuaide, S. (1996). Keeping the wise blood: The construction of images in a mid-life women's group. *Social Work with Groups, 19*(3/4), 131-149.

Montero, I., Ruiz, I., & Hernandez, I. (1993). Social functioning as a significant factor in women's help-seeking behaviour during the climacteric period. *Social Psychiatry and Psychiatric Epidemiology, 28*(4), 178-183.

North American Menopause Society (NAMS). (2001). *Menopause guidebook: Helping women make informed healthcare decisions through perimenopause and beyond.* Cleveland, OH: NAMS.

Pearlman, S. F. (1993). Late mid-life astonishment: Disruption to identity and self-esteem. *Women & Therapy, 14*(1/2) 1-11.

Primomo, J., Yates, B. C., & Woods, N. F. (1990). Social support for women during chronic illness: The relationship among sources and types to adjustment. *Research in Nursing & Health, 13*, 153-161.

Quinio, B. A. (1999). *Women's satisfaction with their health care providers during the menopausal transition.* Unpublished honor's thesis. The Pennsylvania State University, University Park, PA.

Schwarzer, R., & Leppin, A. (1991). Social support and health: A theoretical and empirical overview. *Journal of Social and Personal Relationships, 8*, 99-127.

Shaw, J. (1994). Aging and sexual potential. *Journal of Sex Education and Therapy, 20*, 134-139.

Shumaker, S. A., & Hill, D. R. (1991). Gender differences in social support and physical health. *Health Psychology, 10*, 102-111.

Solomon, L. J., & Rothblum, E. D. (1986). Stress, coping, and social support in women. *The Behavior Therapist, 9*(10), 199-204.

Thoits, P. (1986). Explaining distributions of psychological vulnerability: Lack of social support in the face of life stress. *Social Forces, 63*, 453-481.

Thurau, D. A. (1996). *The relationship between body image and sexuality among menopausal women.* Unpublished master's thesis. The Pennsylvania State University, University Park, PA.

Treloar, A. (1981). Menstrual cyclicity and the perimenopause. *Maturitas, 3*, 249-264.

Uchino, B. N., Cacioppo, J. T., & Kiecolt-Glaser, J. K. (1996). The relationship between social support and physiological processes: A review with emphasis on underlying mechanisms and implication for health. *Psychological Bulletin, 119*, 488-531.

United States Department of Commerce, Bureau of the Census. (1998). *Statistical abstract of the United States: The national data book.* Washington, DC: Bureau of the Census.

Voda, A., & Mansfield, P. K. (1991, June). *Menstrual interval and bleeding changes during the perimenopause.* Paper presented at the 9th meeting of the Society for Menstrual Cycle Research, Seattle, WA.

Walter, C. A. (2000). The psychosocial meaning of menopause: Women's experiences. *Journal of Women & Aging, 12*(3/4), 117-131.

Whittle, G. C., Slade, P., & Ronalds, C. M. (1987). Social support in women reporting dysmenorrhea. *Journal of Psychosomatic Research, 31*, 79-84.

Wilt, C., & Kirk, M. (1995). Menopause: A developmental stage, not a deficiency disease. *Psychotherapy, 32*, 233-241.

BOOK REVIEWS

IS MENSTRUATION OBSOLETE? Coutinho, E. M. and S. J. Segal. *New York: Oxford University Press, 1999.*

This book was originally published in 1996 in Portuguese by the Brazilian gynecologist Elsimar Coutinho, under the title *Menstruation: A Useless Bleeding.* With co-author Sheldon Segal, the book has been revised and translated into English. The book promotes the idea that menstruation is a harmful artifact of modernity and should be suppressed by continuous use of oral contraceptives (OC). Initially, this is advocated mainly for current OC users. Later, they adopt the language of choice and suggest that any woman should be allowed to choose this option. At the end, the authors make it clear that they hope to herald a new paradigm that menstruation is obsolete except when seeking pregnancy.

The authors are medical researchers who specialize in pharmaceutical contraception. Coutinho discovered the contraceptive effects of Depo-Provera and Segal developed Norplant. Both products interfere with regular menstrual bleeding. Coutinho works at a university, and Segal works for the Population Council, a nonprofit research organization that develops and distributes contraception to women in the developing world. They are well-published and established scientists.

The book contains a surprisingly broad range of styles. There are long sections of historical narrative and hypothetical descriptions of prehistoric women's lives. In other sections, it reads like a medical textbook, outlining medical situations and potential treatments. The common thread is a steadfast and unrelenting conviction that menstruation is useless and unnecessary. Anyone who believes otherwise is outdated and misguided.

A book authored by scientists could be expected to be meticulously documented. A reader, however, will be surprised at the difficulty she may have in verifying the claims made by this book. There are no footnotes, and the bibliographic essays at the end of the book often refer to secondary sources. There is no clear link between assertions in the text and the bibliographic materials. For example, we were surprised by the statement that:

http://www.haworthpress.com/store/product.asp?sku=J015
10.1300/J015v27n03_14
195

A 1998 study by the U.S. National Sleep Foundation found that 71 percent
of women reported that their sleep was disturbed in the premenstrual
days and during the first few days of their periods. On average, women
reported that menstruation disrupted their sleep two or three days each
month. (p. 68)

We have not observed this pattern in the hundreds of cycles of daily diary data
that women have collected with us. However, the authors do not provide a reference to this study.

In their efforts to pathologize the menstrual cycle, Coutinho and Segal
make some remarkable claims. They argue that the benefits of suppressing
menstruation extend beyond a woman herself and into her community.
Readers are invited to consider the impact of menstruation on a woman's children and on her productivity as an employee. Through the cost of treating ane-
mia, menstruation endangers public health in the developing world. PMS is
now inflated to include all premenstrual events, even those that a woman herself does not notice.

We now know PMS is biological in nature, and laboratory and neurological tests can record some of these premenstrual events even if they are
barely noticed or perceptible to a woman. (p. 67)

This is quite a change from the days when premenstrual symptoms were dis-
missed as "all in your head." Of course, they argue that PMS is best treated
with continuous OC.

The second platform of Coutinho and Segal's argument is that menstruation
is a *modern* anomaly and that today's women only menstruate because they are
no longer constantly pregnant or breastfeeding. We are not convinced. At the
heart of these arguments is the mistaken belief that a woman who is menstruating regularly must also be ovulating regularly. Ovulatory disturbances are
common, and often occur at the same time as women continue to have menstrual flow at regular, unremarkable intervals (Prior, Vigna, Schecter, & Burgess, 1990). The stresses that disturbed ovulation in prehistoric women were
probably different from those that operate today, but the response of ovulation
to stress was probably similar. Finally, compared with other animals, humans
are not very fertile, so women may continue to menstruate for many cycles before conceiving.

Menstrual cycles do not leave fossil records, but we can learn from women
who live in preindustrial societies today. Women in industrial societies do live
longer, start menstruating earlier, have better control over fertility, and better
nutrition. Dogon women, from an agricultural tribe in Africa, do have fewer
menstrual cycles in a lifetime (estimates are 160 menstrual cycles, just over 12
years) (Strassmann & Warner, 1998). Menstrual cycles are more common today, but they are not a new phenomenon. This is confirmed by a modern

ethnographic study of the !Kung woman Nisa (Shostak, 1981). Nisa, as a young girl, knew that when her mother's periods stopped, she was pregnant.

IS MENSTRUATION AN ORAL CONTRACEPTIVE DEFICIENCY DISEASE?

The idea that women can safely suppress menstruation with daily oral contraceptive use over long periods of time (long OC) has a life beyond this book and needs to be addressed in its own right. We do not believe that government regulating agencies, physicians, or women currently have enough information about the effects of long OC to make a decision about safety. We are also cautious because there is a clear profit motive to promoting the use of OC by all women. Finally, women are vulnerable to exploitation because of the cultural distaste for menstruation (Laws, 1990). From a marketing perspective, the timing of this translation is interesting. A new birth control pill called Seasonale, which is taken daily for many days, is soon to be released. The inventor hopes to gain as much as 20% of the 1.6 billion dollar annual market for oral contraceptives (Anonymous, 2000).

APPROPRIATE TESTING OF "LONG ORAL CONTRACEPTIVES" (LONG OC)

Conventional OC were initially tested solely for their contraceptive effectiveness. Perhaps in the 1950s regulators were unaware that in the 1990s nearly 90% of young women would use them for an average of 6 premenopausal years (Prior et al., 2001). They certainly were ignorant of how high and harmful estrogen levels were in initial OC. The governmental pharmaceutical regulatory bodies that originally allowed OC onto the markets ignored the effects of supra-physiological doses of synthetic ovarian hormones on every tissue of the body. Although we agree that contraception aids are needed to support a woman's control of her fertility, we believe that those regulatory decisions were short-sighted. For example, it is now clear that the first generation of high dose OC put healthy young women at risk for blood clots, strokes, and hypertension (Meade, 1988). The issue of whether OC use increases breast cancer risk has not yet been resolved, although evidence suggests that, like lower dose ovarian steroids given as "replacement" after menopause, breast cancer risk increases (Writing Group for WHI, 2002) particularly for women with a family history of breast cancer (Grabrick et al., 2000). Further, there is a trend over the last 5 decades for a population increase in estrogen-receptor positive breast cancers that may reflect exposure to high dose exogenous estrogen through OC. Although most clinicians believe OC are "good for bones," recent epidemiological data show lower baseline bone mineral density (BMD) values in women who have ever used OC compared to those who haven't (Prior et al., 2001). Epidemiological data also relate OC use to increased fracture rates (Cooper, Hanaford, Croft, & Kay, 1993; Vessey, Mant, & Painter, 1998). In short, although we now know that OC use does not increase mortality (Beral et al., 1999) and does significantly decrease ovarian cancer, it may increase risks for breast cancer and osteoporosis.

It is common to assume that ovarian hormonal effects are restricted to reproductive organs and processes. However, estrogen and progesterone affect tissues throughout the body. There is surprisingly little information on patterns of ovulation and hormone levels during a healthy woman's lifetime. Nor is there adequate information on the long-term health effects of women's own hormonal rhythms. Already only a minority of premenopausal women in Canada have never used OC. We are losing the chance to investigate the epidemiology of natural variation in women's cycles.

LONG OC USE AND NORMAL DEVELOPMENT

One concern is the effect of long OC use on normal developmental processes following menarche. There has been little research on the effects of OC use during the developmental changes of menarche. OC use overwhelms endogenous hormonal signals. Could OC use during puberty affect women decades later during the menopausal transition? Possibly yes. In current use, OC are interrupted for 7 days per month. How important is this hormone-free window to development of a normal self-regulating system? Maturation often involves a critical feedback window. We don't know, but it seems possible that long OC may influence women's reproductive maturation.

Therefore, we believe that the federal Drug Administration in the USA and the Health Protection Branch in Canada must require that long OC be tested for safety prior to marketing. Randomized, double-blind, placebo-controlled testing should take into account the effect of continuous, long OC on bone, endometrium, breasts, and the cardiovascular system. It should also enroll women at different life stages: as young women within 5 years of menarche, premenopausal women, and women in perimenopause. These studies should also monitor women's feelings and experiences with a daily diary self-report instrument (including feelings of frustration, depression, self-worth, energy, anxiety, as well as fluid retention, spotting, migraine headaches, and breast tenderness). Safety monitoring must also follow women after they stop taking long OC to measure how long it takes to initiate normal ovulatory cycles. Finally, because some women experience premenstrual exacerbation of epileptic seizures and migraine headaches, long OC must be placebo-tested in these susceptible women.

CONTRACEPTION AND HUMAN RIGHTS

It is a fundamental right for women to have access to effective contraception and control of reproduction. However, significant human rights violations have been uncovered, both in the initial testing and in more recent distribution of pharmaceutical contraception. Coutinho and Segal cannot be unaware of feminist concerns that women in psychiatric institutions have been forced to use Norplant or Depo-Provera and about the questionable promotion of these methods in the developing world. OC at least can be stopped without the intervention of a health care provider.

THE CULTURAL CONTEXT: LOWER STATUS OF WOMEN AND DENIGRATION OF NATURAL PHYSIOLOGY

This book has been widely publicized because it says in a new way what our culture believes: women's menstruation is smelly, painful, disruptive, and in short, negative. Western culture has viewed women's reproductive system as abnormal and deficient primarily because it differs from men's. This negative view is a self-fulfilling prophecy. If we ask why menstruation is sometimes distasteful, symptomatic, and abnormal, as Coutinho and Segal assert, the primary answer is the lower status of women in society.

The word menstruation means something diametrically different to the authors than it means to us. Menses in an ovulatory cycle are no more objectionable than changing the diaper of a breast-fed baby. The smell is salty and clean, the flow is modest, and often is accompanied by predictable premenstrual symptoms and some cramping. The authors are talking about menstruation from non-ovulatory cycles with high estrogen levels in which the flow is flooding with clots, smells like spoiled fish, is preceded by PMS, and accompanied by severe cramps. We agree that abnormal, non-ovulatory menstruation is unnecessary and should be obsolete!

In addition, ovulation is vulnerable. Ovulation disturbances commonly occur during the first 9 months (on average) after standard OC are discontinued (Bracken, Hellenbrand, & Holford, 1990). School stress can alter both ovulation and menstrual cycle intervals in young women students (Nagata, Kato, Seki, & Furuya, 1986). During the 12 years after the first menstrual period, and in the years leading up to the last menstrual period, ovulation is less consistent than during the premenopausal years (Vollman, 1977). The ovulation disturbances in adolescence and perimenopause seem to be part of the natural pattern of development. In adolescence, ovulatory disturbances are probably only a concern if the young woman is also inactive, overweight, and subject to social stress. During the menopausal transition, ovulation disturbances (often coupled with high estradiol levels) (Prior, 1998) are common (Prior, 2002; Santoro, Rosenberg, Adel, & Skurnick, 1996). Ovulation disturbances in women during the mid-reproductive years are strongly related to the prevalent cultural demand that women be thin. This demand for low weight translates itself for some women into cognitive dietary restraint (worry that eating a particular food will cause obesity). Cognitive dietary restraint is a common psychological stress, disturbs ovulation in women of normal weight, and is associated with high cortisol levels (McLean, Barr, & Prior, 2001a). Cognitive dietary restraint probably causes ovulation disturbances in healthy women (Barr, Janelle, & Prior, 1994; Barr, Prior, & Vigna, 1994). It has also been associated with negative bone changes despite exercise in university students (McLean, Barr, & Prior, 2001b).

Traditionally Medicine (as a sociohistorical entity) and Obstetrics and Gynecology (as a surgical subspecialty devoted to women's pelvic organs) have considered themselves to be the legitimate holders of knowledge about and power over women's reproduction–menopause, pregnancy, and menstruation. All three are prime targets for control. It is not surprising that menstruation is a new frontier for the control of women. This is manifested clearly in the misogyny of *Is Menstruation Obsolete?*

STRATEGIES OTHER THAN LONG OC TO TREAT OR PREVENT ABNORMAL MENSTRUATION

Certainly there are circumstances in which abnormal menstruation should be treated for health. However, there are many strategies to treat abnormal menstruation, and all of them are more physiological and less potentially harmful than long OC. First, we need more data on the prospective epidemiology of ovulation. This accurate information needs to be taught to young women in a positive, woman-affirming context. Second, menstrual cramps can be eliminated and flow decreased by use of anti-prostaglandin medications (e.g., ibuprofen). Third, for women with anovulatory androgen excess (aka polycystic ovary syndrome), replacement of progesterone/progestin that is missing (Prior, 1997) and the addition of spironolactone as an anti-androgen will improve cycles and reduce acne and excess hair. For women with hypothalamic ovulation disturbances, cyclic therapy with progesterone or progestin and the daily diary recording and reframing of negative ideas about menstruation are associated with a 50% one-year recovery rate (Prior, Vigna, Barr, Rexworthy, & Lentle, 1994). Premenstrual symptoms are decreased by mild and increasing exercise (Prior, Vigna, Alojado, Sciarretta, & Schulzer, 1987). Symptoms are also improved by cyclic progesterone (Dennerstein, Spencer-

Gardner, Gotts, Brown, & Smith, 1985) and supplemental calcium (Thys-Jacobs, Starkey, Bernstein, Tian, & Group, 1998).

In puberty when ovulation is being established, cyclic progesterone therapy may not immediately lead to normally ovulatory cycles but will provide normal physiology. In perimenopause, when hypothalamic-pituitary-ovarian feedback is disturbed (Prior, 1998), cyclic progesterone, often in high doses, will control heavy flow, night sweats, and some of the other unwanted symptoms of the menopausal transition.

Effective contraception is an important component of health for women, and oral contraceptives are very effective. Complications from pregnancy are a major source of mortality for women under age 25, particularly women with poor access to medical care. Controlling family size is necessary for a woman's quality of life. However, women do have other choices. One important choice that the authors of this book do not mention is "the morning after pill." This emergency contraception method involves taking several oral contraceptive pills immediately (and again 12 hours later) within 72 hours following a rape or a barrier method failure, and it is available, well-tolerated, and effective (Glaiser, 1997).

Is it safe to suppress menstruation with long-term, continuous oral contraceptives? We do not believe that the data are currently available to decide. There are safer ways to reduce menstruation-related discomfort. There is a great deal of money to be made from the current OC user market, and even more money potentially from women who dislike menstruation and do not need contraception. As baby boom women pass through the perimenopausal transition, OC are touted (with little data) to control heavy bleeding–this is another large potential market.

In summary, this book is not a balanced, scientific consideration of the issues, but rather a polemic against menstruation. Exaggeration is frequent, and it is difficult (or impossible) to verify the claims made in the text. Menstruation with ovulation is an important physiological part of women's lives. It is neither detrimental nor obsolete.

Reviewed by Christine L. Hitchcock and Jerilynn C. Prior

NOTE

Christine L. Hitchcock, PhD, is a research associate and Jerilynn C. Prior, MD, FRCPC, is Professor of Endocrinology at the University of British Columbia. Dr. Prior directs the Centre for Menstrual Cycle and Ovulation Research.

REFERENCES

Anonymous. (2000, July 10). *EVMS begins clinical trials of new birth control concept.* Available at *http://www.evms.edu/about/news/07-10-00.html* (retrieved Sept. 5, 2000).

Barr, S. I., Janelle, K. C., & Prior, J. C. (1994). Vegetarian versus nonvegetarian diets, dietary restraint, and subclinical ovulatory disturbances: Prospective 6 month study. *American Journal of Clinical Nutrition, 60,* 887-894.

Barr, S. I., Prior, J. C., & Vigna, Y. M. (1994). Restrained eating and ovulatory disturbances: Possible implications for bone health. *American Journal of Clinical Nutrition, 59,* 92-97.

Beral, V., Hermon, C., Kay, C., Hannaford, P., Darby, S., & Reeves, G. (1999). Mortality associated with contraceptive use: 25 year follow up of cohort of 46,000 women from Royal College of General Practitioners' oral contraceptive study. *British Medical Journal, 318,* 96-100.

Bracken, H. B., Hellenbrand, K. G., & Holford, T. R. (1990). Conception delay after oral contraceptive use: The effect of estrogen dose. *Fertility and Sterility, 53,* 21-27.

Cooper, C., Hannaford, P., Croft, P., & Kay, C. R. (1993). Oral contraceptive pill use and fractures in women: A prospective study. *Bone, 14,* 41-45.

Dennerstein, L., Spencer-Gardner, C., Gotts, G., Brown, J. B., & Smith, M. A. (1985). Progesterone and the premenstrual syndrome: A double blind crossover trial. *British Medical Journal, 290,* 1617-1621.

Glaiser, A. (1997). Emergency postcoital contraception. *New England Journal of Medicine, 337,* 1058-1064.

Grabick, D. M., Hartmann, L. C., Cerhan, J. R., Vierkant, R. A., Therneau, T. M., Vachon, C. M., Olson, J. E., Couch, F. J., Anderson, K. E., Pankratz, V. S., & Sellers, T. A. (2000). Risk of breast cancer with oral contraceptive use in women with a family history of breast cancer. *Journal of the American Medical Association, 284,* 1791-1798.

Laws, S. (1990). *Issues of blood: The politics of menstruation.* London: MacMillan.

McLean, J. A., Barr, S. I., & Prior, J. C. (2001a). Cognitive dietary restraint is associated with higher urinary cortisol excretion in healthy premenopausal women. *American Journal of Clinical Nutrition, 73,* 7-12.

McLean, J. A., Barr, S. I., & Prior, J. C. (2001b). Dietary restraint, exercise, and bone density in young women: Are they related? *Medicine and Science in Sport and Exercise, 33,* 1292-1296.

Meade, T. W. (1988). Update: Cardiovascular effects of oral contraception and hormonal replacement therapy. *American Journal of Obstetrics and Gynecology, 158,* 1646-1652.

Nagata, I., Kato, K., Seki, K., & Furuya, K. (1986). Ovulatory disturbances: Causative factors among Japanese student nurses in a dormitory. *Journal of Adolescent Health Care, 7,* 1-5.

Prior, J. C. (1997, February). Ovulatory disturbances: They do matter. *Canadian Journal of Diagnosis,* pp. 64-80.

Prior, J. C. (1998). Perimenopause: The complex endocrinology of the menopausal transition. *Endocrine Reviews, 19,* 397-428.

Prior, J. C. (2002). The ageing female reproductive axis II: Ovulatory changes with perimenopause. In J. D. Veldhuis & Z. Laron (Eds.), *Endocrine facets of ageing in the human and experimental animal* (pp. 172-192). London: Wiley.

Prior, J. C., Kirkland, S., Joseph, L., Kreiger, N., Hanley, D. A., Adachi, J. D., Vigna, Y. M., Berger, M. S., Blondeau, L., Jackson, S. A., & Tenenhouse, A. (2001). Oral contraceptive agent use and bone mineral density in premenopausal women: Cross-sectional population-based data from the Canadian Multicentre Osteoporosis Study. *Canadian Medical Association Journal, 165*, 1023-1029.

Prior, J. C., Vigna, Y. M., Alojado, N., Sciaretta, D., & Schulzer, M. (1987). Conditioning exercise decreases premenstrual symptoms: A prospective controlled 6 month trial. *Fertility and Sterility, 47*, 402-408.

Prior, J. C., Vigna, Y. M., Barr, S. I., Rexworthy, C., & Lentle, B. C. (1994). Cyclic medroxyprogesterone treatment increases bone density: A controlled trial in active women with menstrual cycle disturbances. *American Journal of Medicine, 96*, 521-530.

Prior, J. C., Vigna, Y. M., Schecter, M. T., & Burgess, A. E. (1990). Spinal bone loss and ovulatory disturbances. *New England Journal of Medicine, 323*, 1221-1227.

Santoro, N., Rosenberg, J., Adel, T., & Skurnick, J. H. (1996). Characterization of reproductive hormonal dynamics in the perimenopause. *Journal of Clinical Endocrinology and Metabolism, 81*, 1495-1501.

Shostak, M. (1981). *Nisa: The life and words of a !Kung woman*. New York: Vintage Books.

Strassman, B. I., & Warner, J. H. (1998). Predictors of fecundability and conception waits among the Dogon of Mali. *American Journal of Physical Anthropology, 105*, 167-184.

Thys-Jacob, S., Starkey, P., Bernstein, D., Tian, J., & Group, T. P. (1998). Calcium carbonate and the premenstrual syndrome: Effects on premenstrual and menstrual symptoms. *American Journal of Obstetrics and Gynecology, 179*, 444-452.

Vessey, M., Mant, J., & Painter, R. (1998). Oral contraception and other factors in relation to hospital referral for fracture: Findings in a large cohort study. *Contraception, 57*, 231-235.

Vollman, R. F. (1977). The menstrual cycle. In E. A. Friedman (Ed.), *Major problems in obstetrics and gynecology* (vol. 1, pp. 11-93). Toronto: Saunders.

Writing Group for WHI. (2002). Risks and benefits of estrogen plus progestin in healthy postmenopausal women: Principal results from the Women's Health Initiative randomized controlled trial. *Journal of the American Medical Association, 288*, 321-333.

THE CURSE: CONFRONTING THE LAST UNMENTIONABLE TABOO–
MENSTRUATION. Houppert, K. *New York: Farrar, Straus, & Giroux, 1999.*

The Curse is a well-researched, intriguing compilation of information about
menstruation from journal articles, advice columns, news reports, advertisements for feminine hygiene products, focus groups, magazine articles, books,
movies, and public relations campaigns. The tone of the book is humorous yet
stern, and the author strategically mixes personal experiences and historical
facts. Houppert is a journalist who uses her investigative skills to present a "be-
hind the scenes" look at political and cultural messages about menstruation,
sexuality, PMS, and menopause. *The Curse* is divided into four sections: the
industry, the adolescent, the adult, and the menstrual subculture.

In the first section, Houppert reviews the motivations of the 8 billion dollar
menstrual products industry. She examines how "our culture conspires to
transform monthly bleeding from a benign inconvenience into a shameful, embarrassing and even debilitating event" (p. 10). Houppert playfully wrote,
"Blood is kinda like snot. How come it's not treated that way?" (p. 4). Fear of
discovery fuels the menstrual products industry. If girls and women are
ashamed of menstruation, they will pay for products that conceal monthly
flow.

Houppert discusses the research on dioxin poisoning from tampon use and
the lack of public knowledge about these risks. She states that despite findings
that support the link between tampons and the toxic effects of dioxin, the industry claims that dioxin found in their products is not a health threat. Are they
simply naïve? It's more likely that the industry would prefer that the data about
dioxin were not publicized because they risk losing consumers and would need
to invest in research on alternative materials for tampons.

The second section contains information about adolescents' experiences
with menarche, their sources of information about it, and cultural stereotypes
about menstruating women. Houppert's interviews with 9-10-year-old girls
reveal the importance of concealment, a lack of knowledge, and the prevalence
of myths about menstruation. She found that girls are curious about menstruation; however, they have little knowledge about the menstrual cycle. We need
more open discussions about menstruation in order to refute myths about menstruation and help girls feel comfortable about their bodies and their emerging
sexuality.

In the third section, Houppert focuses on adults' experiences with menstruation. She gives an historical account of Premenstrual Syndrome (PMS) from
1878 to today's culturally accepted concept of PMS as an excuse for women's
anger and moodiness. The medicalization and socialization of PMDD and
PMS are discussed. Houppert concludes that the major theme in PMS literature is that women are afraid of feeling "out of control."

The final section challenges the culture of concealment of menstruation. Houppert found only three adult resources that attempt to reframe attitudes toward and education about menstruation: a new menstrual products company (InSync Miniforms), a collection of goddess-feminists who celebrate their cycles, and the Museum of Menstruation. InSync Miniforms are pad-tampon hybrids that are held in place by a woman's own anatomy. The goddess-feminists hope to "reclaim a time when the feminine cycle was integrated into our common experience of life" (pp. 215-216). The Museum of Menstruation (MUM) is Harry Finley's personal collection of menstrual paraphernalia. His collection is both virtual (http://www.mum.org) and real (displayed in the basement of Finley's house). He has had many visitors to his museum, and he is an enthusiastic one-man movement for openness and education.

Houppert conveys a witty understanding of the history, politics, and socialization of menstruation. The Curse is enlightening, thought-provoking, and accessible. Houppert's extensive critique of the menstrual products industry is as fascinating as Jean Kilbourne's analysis of the diet industry. I would recommend The Curse to anyone interested in women's health. It is ideal for researchers and women's studies classes. It's also an excellent resource for therapists who work with adolescents; however, parts of the book are too advanced for younger girls to comprehend. The Curse is a critique of the sociocultural aspects of menstruation. Houppert leaves readers wondering, "Why don't we just treat menstruation like the common cold?" (p. 243).

Reviewed by Jennifer Gorman Rose

NOTE

Jennifer Gorman Rose, MA, is a full-time lecturer in psychology at Connecticut College. She is a member of the Society for Menstrual Cycle Research, and she has presented the results of her research on women's menarche stories, educational pamphlets about menstruation, and the socialization of menstruation.

BEFORE SHE GETS HER PERIOD: TALKING WITH YOUR DAUGHTER ABOUT MENSTRUATION. Gillooly, J. B. *Los Angeles: Perspective Publishing, 1998.*

PERIOD: A GIRL'S GUIDE. Loulan, J. and B. Worthen. *Minnetonka, MN: Book Peddlers, 2001.*

Many mothers dread the responsibility of explaining menstruation to their daughters. When is the right time to begin such a discussion? How will I know when she's ready? What does she know already and what information does she need from me? What if she seems embarrassed or disinterested? Gillooly's *Before She Gets Her Period: Talking with Your Daughter About Menstruation* addresses these concerns and provides the encouragement that some mothers may need in order to begin a dialogue with their young daughters about menstruation.

Although the biological basics are covered, the emphasis of this book is on the emotional implications of menarche. Gillooly encourages mothers to recall their own first period in order to better relate to their daughter's feelings and concerns. In fact, all of the advice and wisdom in this book is supplemented with firsthand accounts from young girls, adult women looking back on their first periods, and even fathers and brothers recounting their experiences when their daughters and sisters began menstruation.

One of the most unique and valuable features of this book is its emphasis on the influence of culture on attitudes toward menstruation. The suggestion is that when mothers openly talk with their daughters about menstruation, they will help them to view it as a natural process and a rite of passage. Gillooly suggests planning some type of ritual, maybe a special dinner or evening out, to celebrate the beginning of a daughter's transition to adulthood.

Tips about how much to cover in one sitting, what type of information is most valuable to young girls, and how to handle emotional outbursts are included. Common fears, such as having "it" arrive while at school, are also addressed. What is most emphasized, though, is the importance of beginning this sort of dialogue early. Establishing open communication is important during preadolescence, but will be even more valuable as daughters mature and face bigger and more difficult challenges.

Gillooly also encourages open discussion with boys and men. This is especially important to fathers who will want to learn how to relate to their adolescent daughters and to brothers who are inherently curious and want to be included. Teaching boys about menstruation and including them in this way may discourage the teasing that many young girls face and may encourage bonding between brothers and sisters.

Despite the encouragement and supportive tone of Gillooly's book, some mothers may still believe that they need an easier way to begin a dialogue about menstruation. For these mothers, a basic book written for girls may be a good starting point. *Period: A Girl's Guide* provides practical information for the young girl who is anticipating her first menstrual period. Loulan and Worthen have provided a comprehensive guide to the menstrual cycle in language that is accessible to the average 8-12-year-old girl. This "child-friendly" resource is filled with delightful line drawings and information that is presented in a straightforward, yet supportive manner.

In addition to the biological explanation of the menstrual cycle, practical issues such as how to use menstrual management products and what to expect emotionally are addressed. A brief description of what goes on during a pelvic exam is also included to take some of the mystery and fear out of a girl's first visit to the gynecologist. *Period* is a good beginner's source of accurate information about menstruation and the related issues of body image and self-esteem.

Although technical and practical information remain important, what makes this book special is its emphasis on the wide range of experiences that are considered normal. The authors reassure girls that it is normal for some women to experience menstrual cramps and for some others to have painless periods. Readers are reminded that some women experience mood changes, but others do not. The individuality of each girl is celebrated throughout the text and in the illustrations.

The physical and psychological changes that come with the onset of menstruation can be both confusing and stressful. Knowledge can help to ease this transition. Whether mothers choose to provide their daughters with an introductory book or to take on the task of explaining menstruation themselves, preparing young girls emotionally by providing them with an idea of what to expect is what matters most. Both *Period* and *Before She Gets Her Period* can be helpful tools for mothers who must take on this important task.

Reviewed by Elyse A. Warren

NOTE

Elyse A. Warren is a doctoral candidate in educational psychology at Teachers College, Columbia University and a lecturer in the Department of Psychology at Connecticut College.

Index

Refugee Women and Their Mental Health: Shattered Societies, Shattered Lives, edited by Ellen Cole, PhD, Oliva M. Espin, PhD, and Esther D. Rothblum, PhD (Vol. 13, No. 1/2/3, 1992). *"The ideas presented are rich and the perspectives varied, and the book is an important contribution to understanding refugee women in a global context." (Contemporary Psychology)*

Women, Girls and Psychotherapy: Reframing Resistance, edited by Carol Gilligan, PhD, Annie Rogers, PhD, and Deborah Tolman, EdD (Vol. 11, No. 3/4, 1991). *"Of use to educators, psychotherapists, and parents–in short, to any person who is directly involved with girls at adolescence." (Harvard Educational Review)*

Professional Training for Feminist Therapists: Personal Memoirs, edited by Esther D. Rothblum, PhD, and Ellen Cole, PhD (Vol. 11, No. 1, 1991). *"Exciting, interesting, and filled with the angst and the energies that directed these women to develop an entirely different approach to counseling." (Science Books & Films)*

Jewish Women in Therapy: Seen But Not Heard, edited by Rachel Josefowitz Siegel, MSW, and Ellen Cole, PhD (Vol. 10, No. 4, 1991). *"A varied collection of prose and poetry, first-person stories, and accessible theoretical pieces that can help Jews and non-Jews, women and men, therapists and patients, and general readers to grapple with questions of Jewish women's identities and diversity." (Canadian Psychology)*

Women's Mental Health in Africa, edited by Esther D. Rothblum, PhD, and Ellen Cole, PhD (Vol. 10, No. 3, 1990). *"A valuable contribution and will be of particular interest to scholars in women's studies, mental health, and cross-cultural psychology." (Contemporary Psychology)*

Motherhood: A Feminist Perspective, edited by Jane Price Knowles, MD, and Ellen Cole, PhD (Vol. 10, No. 1/2, 1990). *"Provides some enlightening perspectives. . . . It is worth the time of both male and female readers." (Contemporary Psychology)*

Diversity and Complexity in Feminist Therapy, edited by Laura Brown, PhD, ABPP, and Maria P. P. Root, PhD (Vol. 9, No. 1/2, 1990). *"A most convincing discussion and illustration of the importance of adopting a multicultural perspective for theory building in feminist therapy. . . . This book is a must for therapists and should be included on psychology of women syllabi." (Association for Women in Psychology Newsletter)*

Fat Oppression and Psychotherapy, edited by Laura S. Brown, PhD, and Esther D. Rothblum, PhD (Vol. 8, No. 3, 1990). *"Challenges many traditional beliefs about being fat . . . A refreshing new perspective for approaching and thinking about issues related to weight." (Association for Women in Psychology Newsletter)*

Lesbianism: Affirming Nontraditional Roles, edited by Esther D. Rothblum, PhD, and Ellen Cole, PhD (Vol. 8, No. 1/2, 1989). *"Touches on many of the most significant issues brought before therapists today." (Newsletter of the Association of Gay & Lesbian Psychiatrists)*

Women and Sex Therapy: Closing the Circle of Sexual Knowledge, edited by Ellen Cole, PhD, and Esther D. Rothblum, PhD (Vol. 7, No. 2/3, 1989). *"Adds immeasureably to the feminist therapy literature that dispels male paradigms of pathology with regard to women." (Journal of Sex Education & Therapy)*

The Politics of Race and Gender in Therapy, edited by Lenora Fulani, PhD (Vol. 6, No. 4, 1988). *Women of color examine newer therapies that encourage them to develop their historical identity.*

Treating Women's Fear of Failure, edited by Esther D. Rothblum, PhD, and Ellen Cole, PhD (Vol. 6, No. 3, 1988). *"Should be recommended reading for all mental health professionals, social workers, educators, and vocational counselors who work with women." (The Journal of Clinical Psychiatry)*

Women, Power, and Therapy: Issues for Women, edited by Marjorie Braude, MD (Vol. 6, No. 1/2, 1987). *"Raise[s] therapists' consciousness about the importance of considering gender-based power in therapy . . . welcome contribution." (Australian Journal of Psychology)*

Dynamics of Feminist Therapy, edited by Doris Howard (Vol. 5, No. 2/3, 1987). *"A comprehensive treatment of an important and vexing subject." (Australian Journal of Sex, Marriage and Family)*

A Woman's Recovery from the Trauma of War: Twelve Responses from Feminist Therapists and Activists, edited by Esther D. Rothblum, PhD, and Ellen Cole, PhD (Vol. 5, No. 1, 1986). *"A milestone. In it, twelve women pay very close attention to a woman who has been deeply wounded by war." (The World)*

Women and Mental Health: New Directions for Change, edited by Carol T. Mowbray, PhD, Susan Lanir, MA, and Marilyn Hulce, MSW, ACSW (Vol. 3, No. 3/4, 1985). *"The overview of sex differences in disorders is clear and sensitive, as is the review of sexual exploitation of clients by therapists. . . . Mandatory reading for all therapists who work with women." (British Journal of Medical Psychology and The British Psychological Society)*

Women Changing Therapy: New Assessments, Values, and Strategies in Feminist Therapy, edited by Joan Hamerman Robbins and Rachel Josefowitz Siegel, MSW (Vol. 2, No. 2/3, 1983). *"An excellent collection to use in teaching therapists that reflection and resolution in treatment do not simply lead to adaptation, but to an active inner process of judging." (News for Women in Psychiatry)*

Current Feminist Issues in Psychotherapy, edited by The New England Association for Women in Psychology (Vol. 1, No. 3, 1983). *Addresses depression, displaced homemakers, sibling incest, and body image from a feminist perspective.*

Made in the USA
Lexington, KY
04 September 2015